Ea
Los

By the same author

on medicine

The Medicine Men
Paper Doctors
Everything You Want to Know About Ageing
Stress Control
The Home Pharmacy
Aspirin or Ambulance
Face Values
Stress and Your Stomach
Guilt
The Good Medicine Guide
A Guide to Child Health
Bodypower
An A to Z of Women's Problems
Bodysense
Taking Care of Your Skin
Life Without Tranquillisers
High Blood Pressure
Diabetes
Arthritis
Eczema and Dermatitis
The Story of Medicine
Natural Pain Control
Mindpower
Addicts and Addictions
Dr Vernon Coleman's Guide to Alternative Medicine
Stress Management Techniques
Overcoming Stress
The 20 Minute Health Check
Know Yourself
The Health Scandal
Sex For Everyone
Mind Over Body

on cricket

Thomas Winsden's Cricketing Almanack
Diary of a Cricket Lover

as Edward Vernon

Practice Makes Perfect
Practise What You Preach
Getting Into Practice
Aphrodisiacs – an Owner's Manual
The Complete Guide to Life

as Marc Charbonnier

Tunnel

Eat Green, Lose Weight

How to Slim Successfully the Natural Way

Dr Vernon Coleman

ANGUS
& ROBERTSON
PUBLISHERS

ANGUS & ROBERTSON PUBLISHERS

16 Golden Square, London W1R 4BN
United Kingdom and
Unit 4, Eden Park, 31 Waterloo Road,
North Ryde, NSW, Australia 2113.

First published in the United Kingdom by
Angus & Robertson (UK) in 1990

Copyright © Dr Vernon Coleman 1990

Cover design by Mark Foster, Illustration by Jakki Wood

Typeset in Great Britain by The Wordshop,
Rossendale, Lancs

Printed in Finland

British Library Cataloguing in Publication Data
Coleman, Vernon
Eat green, lose weight
I. Title
613.2'5

ISBN 0 207 16577 7

A GENTLE WARNING

Eating according to the guidelines in this book can only do you good. But do please consult your doctor before changing your eating habits if you are receiving medical attention or if you have any symptoms of illness or problems with your health. There is an excellent chance that if you change your diet your need for medical treatment may change (for example, if you have high blood pressure, arthritis or heart trouble you may be able to cut down or stop drug treatment).

Author's Note

Trying to decide whether or not to buy a book can be difficult. A quick flick through the pages doesn't always tell you whether or not you're really going to benefit. You should buy this book if:

- you would like to get slim – and stay slim – and you're fed up with short-term diets which either fail or become boring
- you'd like to eat a healthy diet – but you're not sure which foods to avoid, and you don't want to have to give up everything you enjoy
- you're thinking about becoming a vegetarian but you've still got some questions you'd like answered – and some doubts and fears that need allaying

If these are subjects which interest you and you want the facts and some plain, straightforward, simple to follow advice then you need *Eat Green – Lose Weight*.

Vernon Coleman

Contents

PART THREE: FOOD AND RECIPES

PART ONE
THE GREEN REVOLUTION

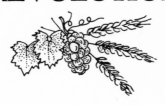

1
Turning Green

The diet that makes sense

Today we ought to be healthier than ever before. We spend more on health care than at any other time in history. We allocate huge sums of money to medical research. Our hospitals are stocked with hi-tech equipment. Our clinics are staffed by well-trained specialists. We use more sophisticated farming techniques than ever before and more advanced food preparation methods and packaging. Large multi-national companies pay out fortunes on attempts to preserve and improve the quality of what we eat.

But not only are we no healthier than our ancestors – the evidence shows that in many ways we have never been sicker. Cancer was virtually unknown in the nineteenth century, but throughout the twentieth its incidence has rocketed. High blood pressure, heart disease and strokes are all far commoner than ever before. The number of diabetics is doubling every ten years. Allergies occur far more frequently, as do indigestion, peptic ulcers and bowel problems of all kinds. Anxiety and depression are commonplace, food poisoning of all sorts is on the increase, and with each new year doctors see more patients suffering from disorders as varied as migraine and arthritis.

Some might choose to claim that we suffer more from diseases such as cancer and heart disease, and from degenerative disorders such as arthritis, because we live much longer than our ancestors. But this argument simply does not stand up to close examination. The truth is that we only *seem* to live longer than the generations which came before us because the number of babies and infants who die today is far smaller than the number who died in more primitive times. A few thousand

– even a few hundred – years ago a massive proportion of babies never reached childhood. These early deaths meant that the *average* life expectation was lower than it is today.

Modern infant mortality rates are comparatively low, but adults live little longer than their counterparts of a century or two ago. It simply isn't possible to explain away our increasing weakness, vulnerability and susceptibility to illness on the grounds that we are living longer. We aren't. So, what has changed? There are a number of possible explanations.

On the surface we may appear to live in a safe and relatively unthreatening world. Theoretically we in the West ought to be more comfortable and contented than any previous generation. We have electricity available at the flick of a switch and running water at the turn of a tap. We have plenty of clothes to keep us warm, and we are surrounded by gadgets designed to make our lives easier and more enjoyable. We can pick up a telephone and talk to friends across the world. Theoretically, we ought to be free of pressure, stress and worry.

But we're not. We are exposed to more stress than any of our ancestors. And we suffer more from stress-related diseases than any of our predecessors did.

The reason for this is simple. The bodies we live in were designed a long, long time ago and were designed for a rather different world – a world of threatening, easily visible enemies, creating immediate problems that required immediate solutions. Our bodies were designed to help us solve physical problems with physical action. If we came face to face with fierce, carnivorous animals our muscles would tighten, our blood pressure would rise, our hearts would beat faster and adrenalin would surge through our veins.

However, our world has changed a lot in the last century or so. We have created a new environment for ourselves. Today our problems are neither simple nor straightforward. Few of them are easily solved with physical action. As a result, stress is now universally recognized as a significant cause of illness and distress.

Pollutants are a major problem, too. Some are environmental – the chemicals which affect the air we breathe and the water we drink, and which commonly come from factories or motor vehicles. Other pollutants are more personal; the most significant of these are, of course, the cancer-producing chemicals which are produced by the smoking of tobacco.

But in addition to these hazards there is now no doubt that one of the most significant causes of illness and early death is the quality of the food we eat. Even though most of us have access to more than enough food, and few citizens of modern, developed countries starve to death these days, the incidence of malnutrition is astonishingly high. The poor quality of our food is undoubtedly one of the major contemporary influences on our health.

There is a simple explanation for this apparent paradox. Although most of us have plenty to eat, much of it has been so thoroughly processed that the constituents from which we prepare our meals would be more accurately described as 'products' than as food. Remarkably, three-quarters of what we eat consists of processed, packaged and heavily refined food. Too often today's food-processing plants remove the essential nutrients from food and replace them with potentially harmful additives. During the last ten years or so numerous researchers around the world have shown that there are close and incontrovertible links between on the one hand the types of food we eat, and on the other the incidence of illness and the accumulation of unwanted fat.

The majority of individuals who have a weight problem get most of their energy – and their calories – from fatty, sugar-rich, heavily refined food. Heart disease, digestive disturbances, high blood pressure, allergies and many other food-related disorders occur more frequently among those who live on a diet of additive-rich, prepared and packaged foods. And as the fat content of meat has become ever higher, so the incidence of specifically fat-related disorders has exploded. Advertising campaigns designed to sell these foods are growing more sophisticated and successful, and as a result the problem is getting worse. While half the world's population is starving to death, the other half suffers from the effects of over-consumption of unnatural food. The evidence shows that the Western world needs to learn to eat more sensibly.

During the 1980's over sixty major reports have been published in many countries by committees who had been given the task of investigating just how dangerous our eating habits have become. Well over three-quarters of those committees recommended that we should eat less fat. The majority suggested that we should eat less sugar. And more than half enthusiastically put forward the idea that we should eat more fibre.

Sadly, these recommendations have not been accepted without opposition from those with a vested interest in the manufacture and sale of additive-rich food. Recently a considerable amount of confusion has been produced – often quite deliberately – by 'experts' paid to support a particular cause. The best example is animal fats. Just about every major scientific and medical committee in the world has agreed that we eat too much butter and too much fatty meat, and drink too much rich, creamy milk. In countries where the fat consumption has fallen (and other factors have remained fairly steady) heart disease rates have also fallen.

But like all evidence linking behaviour to disease, it is largely circumstantial. Scientists cannot prove that fat causes heart disease any more than they can prove that cigarettes cause lung cancer. Despite the agreement of honest, independent experts there must always be a whisper of doubt. And that provides commercial pressure groups with a weakness to exploit. The food industry realized years ago that you can buy any number of apparently reputable medical experts with a few grants and a fistful of airline tickets, and much of the current confusion about food has been created by lobbying paid for by certain aggressive, cash-inspired elements of the industry. It is hardly surprising that few people know what to believe – or what to eat – any more.

The aim of *Eat Green – Lose Weight* is to help you in two ways. First, I want to tell you the truth about food: the truth about fats, protein, carbohydrates, vitamins and minerals; the truth about salt, bread, milk, eggs, meat and all other common foodstuffs; and the truth about the colourants, preservatives and other additives that we consume daily. And second, I want to show you how you can get rid of your bad eating habits and acquire new ones that you'll find easy to keep.

The evidence and advice I have accumulated will help you eat a healthier diet and lose unwanted weight. Most important of all, you will benefit permanently. Because you will have acquired new eating habits you will be able to remain slim and healthy for life. Unlike diets which you might have tried before, you will find my advice easy to follow and easy to stick to. You will succeed because you will enjoy your new eating habits, and because you will feel good about the changes.

You will soon see that my advice makes sense on health grounds. It makes sense on moral grounds. And it makes sense on environmental grounds. You will find that my diet makes it remarkably easy for you to lose weight naturally, inevitably and permanently. Changing your eating habits will give you an excellent opportunity to give up all your bad eating habits and start eating only when you are genuinely hungry. Within months you will feel healthier, fitter, stronger and happier.

It's enough to make you green

A few years ago vegetarians were rare creatures – pitiful figures of fun who were scorned and much abused, harmless but cranky. Female vegetarians were expected to be rather cheerful and weather-burned, friendly rather than feminine. They were widely believed to scorn supporting underwear and to wear dull, dark, floor-length clothes to disguise their shapelessness. Male vegetarians were thought of as bearded, skinny individuals with a penchant for plastic, open-toed sandals, wrinkled, faded corduroy and steel-framed spectacles.

QUESTION: *Isn't a vegetarian diet deadly dull? How can you live on a constant diet of cabbage and lettuce leaves?*

ANSWER: *If you think a vegetarian diet must be dull and boring, that's probably because you've been brought up to regard meat as the only really essential foodstuff and to think of vegetables, fruits, pulses, cereals and so on as being of secondary importance.*

There is no doubt that vegetarian food has had a pretty dire reputation. Even today, many hotels and restaurants get no further than a mushroom omelette and a tomato salad. And the accursed nut cutlet has done much to damage the reputation of vegetarian cooking. The two things that newly converted vegetarians often complain about are a lack of colour and a lack of texture in their food. Both problems are fairly easily solved once you stop thinking of what you're missing (i.e. meat or fish) and start looking at the possibilities.

Try looking around in your local supermarket or greengrocer's at the variety of fruits and vegetables. You'll probably find a dozen things you've never even tasted – or certainly not thought of as having much potential. Cooking – and eating – can be just as exciting and as satisfying without meat as with it.

Things have changed. Vegetarianism is now trendy – particularly among the young, the well-off and the well-educated. The consumption of meat is beginning to fall. One-third of all women have now either completely stopped eating meat or have cut down dramatically. At the same time the consumption of vegetables and fresh fruit has rocketed. Most major supermarkets are beginning to stock a variety of ready-to-cook vegetarian meals, and even fast food chains are catering for the market by selling vegetarian meals. If present trends continue – and all the evidence suggests that they will – then by the year 2000 meat-eaters will, like smokers, be in the minority.

QUESTION: *Is a vegetarian diet more expensive than an ordinary diet?*

ANSWER: *No. If anything it's cheaper. Meat – and meat products – are extremely expensive to buy – and are likely to get even more so in the future.*

There are several reasons why people are giving up meat and becoming vegetarians. First, many people are becoming aware that our modern meat-based, fat-rich diet is not a healthy one. The move away from additive-rich, junk food and towards a healthy, natural diet has been a gradual one, but today most doctors accept that our eating habits are responsible for a considerable amount of disease. It isn't just meat, of course. Biscuits, chocolates, crisps, packaged convenience foods and TV dinners have all come under attack. But meat – and meat products such as hamburgers, sausages and pies – are undoubtedly responsible for many of the commonest ailments which cause illness and early death. Modern farming practices and manufacturing techniques mean that meat products don't only contain huge amounts of fat and other harmful ingredients but are also likely to be contaminated with infective organisms. I shall deal with many of the disorders known to be associated with the consumption of meat on pages 61 – 67.

Second, thousands of people give up meat as they become aware of the cruelty involved in keeping and preparing animals for us to eat – or, for many people, of the simple immorality of breeding animals purely to be eaten. It was this moral worry which led me into becoming a vegetarian.

I live in a beautiful part of the English countryside and my study overlooks our meadow, a three-acre patch of grassland that runs down to a beautifully clear stream. It was spring and the fields nearby were full of milk-heavy sheep and dozens of new-born lambs. Suddenly, I heard the desperate sound of a distraught mother and lamb calling to one another. I got up from my desk and looked out of the window. Somehow a lamb had managed to force its way through the thick bramble hedge that separates our meadow from one of the large fields attached to a nearby farm. I watched as the lamb tried, and failed, to scramble back through the hedge that separated it from its mother.

QUESTION: *Animals kill one another all the time. What's so different about humans killing animals for food?*

ANSWER: *First, some animals are carnivores – they have to eat meat to stay alive. We don't. Second, wild animals usually kill their prey fairly quickly. In contrast many animals kept on farms – and all those killed in abattoirs – are usually treated extremely badly.*

After calling noisily for a couple of minutes the unhappy mother put her head down and followed her lamb into our rather lush-looking stretch of pasture land. Reunited lamb and mother nuzzled one another affectionately. I could be wrong, but I'm prepared to swear that it seemed to me that the lamb got a ticking off for straying so far from home.

You can probably guess what happened next. Once one sheep has found its way through a hedge, every other sheep in the neighbourhood has to follow. Sheep are more curious than cats and more easily led than schoolchildren. Within five minutes our meadow was thick with rather ponderous-looking sheep and a couple of dozen bouncing lambs. I watched them in amazement. I'd never really *watched* lambs at play before. They really do bounce into the air. They really do gambol, play and spring around like happy children. They play tag, hide and seek and all the other simple, old-fashioned playground games. I watched them for an hour.

That evening we went out to dinner with friends at a local restaurant. The first item I saw on the menu was lamb. A few years ago the first thing I would think of if anyone said 'lamb' was 'mint sauce'. But that evening all I could think of were the happy, playful creatures I had seen in our meadow. How on earth could I possibly *eat* a chunk taken out of one of those lambs? I ordered an omelette and have never eaten meat since.

Only afterwards did I discover that I am part of one of the most popular, fashionable and rapidly growing of all trends. This is rather unusual for me, since I have spent most of my life swimming upstream.

Like many people I know, I had for years happily and unquestioningly accepted the curious social rules which make it perfectly acceptable in Britain for pigs, cows and sheep to be killed and chopped up into serving-sized portions, but which make it totally unacceptable for horses (which are certainly no more or less intelligent than pigs and cows) to be treated cruelly or, horror of horrors, to be slaughtered, carved to bits and then eaten with plenty of mustard and two vegetables. I had, I confess with no slight shame, also managed to ignore the fact that most of the animals we eat are kept in obscene conditions, transported in a barbaric way and killed with staggering cruelty and a total lack of compassion. Once I started to ask questions about the way that animals are treated I found it increasingly difficult to defend the disgusting things we pay other people to do on our behalf. In case you remain unconvinced and would like to know more about the way animals are treated on our behalf, I have described the breeding and killing of animals for meat in greater detail on pages 85 – 89.

These two reasons – a concern about health and a moral, emotional anxiety about what we are doing to animals – are the two most common arguments for giving up meat. But they aren't the only reasons why people become vegetarians.

Some people do so because they actually dislike meat or find it too expensive (paradoxically, as the quality of meat has gone down and the number of contaminants has gone up, so the price has increased). Many have stopped eating meat for religious reasons. Several Eastern faiths – notably Hinduism and Buddhism – encourage vegetarianism. Seventh Day Adventists don't eat meat; nor do members of some other branches of Christianity, and many monks.

Others have turned vegetarian because they have become aware that if fewer people in the West ate meat then there would be far less hunger in the world's developing countries.

QUESTION: *Will becoming a vegetarian help me get slim?*

ANSWER: *Yes. Not because meat is rich in calories, but because by changing your eating habits you will be able to get rid of the old, bad habits that helped make you fat and replace them with better, new habits that will help you get slim and stay slim. Becoming a vegetarian means changing your whole way of eating – and, very often, changing the way you think about food too. It means discovering new types of food and new recipes. And it will give you an opportunity to get into the habit of eating only when you are hungry. When I first became a vegetarian I lost over 14lb (6kg) in six months without any effort at all.*

Meat is expensive to produce compared to crops, and the amount of land needed to create one pound of animal protein is considerably greater that that needed to produce one pound of vegetable protein. There is absolutely no doubt that if more people in developed countries ate less meat, and more land was devoted to cereal-growing, then there would be little or no starvation in Africa and Asia.

Finally, a number of people have either given up meat

altogether or cut down their consumption of it so as to lose weight. Vegetarians are far less likely to get fat than meat-eaters, and thousands of slimmers have already found that it is considerably easier to lose weight (and to do so *permanently*) on a vegetarian diet than on a fat-rich meat-containing diet.

Shades of greenness

There are a lot of options open to anyone who wants to eat less meat – there are several acceptable shades of green! Your own personal feelings must decide how green you go, and the speed at which you do it. You do not have to give up all meat and animal products overnight – unless you want to. You must decide what is right for you, how far you want to go and how fast you want to change your eating habits. Choose a lifestyle with which you feel comfortable. And although you may feel that you want to stop eating meat immediately and per-manently, there is nothing wrong with simply cutting down your consumption slowly over a period of time. The route you choose will depend upon your own personal feelings and upon your hopes and expectations. If you want to give up meat because you can't bear the thought of animals being slaught-ered on your behalf, then you will probably want to give up immediately. But if you want to cut down your meat consumption for health reasons or to help you lose weight, you may prefer to change your eating habits slowly.

You need a sense of humour to survive a holiday as a vegetarian. Shortly after I'd become one I booked a skiing holiday in Austria. I told the travel agency and the holiday company that I wanted vegetarian food. However, the hotel staff were desperately confused. They tried hard, but one memorable meal consisted of two spoonsful of mashed potato!

In most areas there are now specialist vegetarian res-taurants, but I firmly believe that all vegetarians should visit as many hotels and restaurants as possible and ask for their kind of food. If enough customers ask, even the most backward-thinking hoteliers and restaurateurs will eventually oblige – for simple commercial reasons. My local fish and chip shop (which cooks in vegetable oil) has started to sell vegetarian burgers in response to my repeated requests for an alternative to fish or sausages. Many fast food chains now serve beanburgers, and some sell baked potatoes with a variety of fillings. And it is possible to have an excellent vegetarian meal from an ordinary Indian or Chinese restaurant.

QUESTION: *If I turn vegetarian, what happens about eating out – when I'm on holiday, or when I go to a restaurant, or if I have to travel by air, or when the family wants a take-away?*

ANSWER: *You'll have some good experiences and some excellent meals, and you'll have some absolute disasters. If you're booking a table at a restaurant do make sure beforehand that they serve vegetarian food; and if you're booking into a hotel take the same precaution. When travelling by air make sure that the airline knows – they'll usually provide you with a vegetarian meal that will probably be better than the meal everyone else gets. If you're going on a package holiday, tell the company – but don't expect them to take any notice.*

You can also get vegetarian food in most hospitals and prisons – though if it's at all possible they do like you to tell them in advance.

If you have to go to dinners where there is a set menu, and haven't been able to arrange an alternative menu for yourself, choose a plain main dish and have plenty of vegetables. If the plate arrives with meat on it – just leave it.

I've eaten at dinners where no one has known that I'm a vegetarian, and to avoid embarrassing my hosts I've simply eaten my way round all the meat dishes unnoticed.

There are four basic stages of vegetarianism. First, as mentioned above, you can simply reduce your meat consumption. Cutting out meat altogether can be difficult: most of us are brought up to regard meat as the central part of any main meal, and psychological dependence on it can be very powerful. Theoretically, of course, someone who eats any meat at all is not a vegetarian, but lowering your meat consumption can be an important step towards improving your health and your figure – as well as making a modest but important statement about the inhumane way that farm animals are treated. Most people who cut down on meat – but

---

don't stop eating it altogether — begin by avoiding fatty cuts, and by having meat only once or twice a week. People who refuse pork, lamb, veal and beef but who do eat poultry and fish are usually known as demi-vegetarians.

Second, you can cut out all meat — including chicken — but continue to eat fish. People who feel uncomfortable about eating meat of any kind but who find it difficult to regard a diet based on vegetables as completely satisfying or wholesome will often pass through a fish-eating stage.

The next stage is full vegetarianism. The real vegetarian eats no meat and no fish but does eat animal products such as eggs, milk and cheese. (Strictly speaking, vegetarians who eat both eggs and dairy products are known as lacto-ovo-vegetarians, while people who give up eggs but continue to eat dairy products are known as lacto-vegetarians. I think these subdivisions are rather irrelevant and unnecessary, but I mention them because you will probably hear them used at some time or other.)

The final step is to become a vegan. A true vegan does not eat any animal products at all — no eggs, no cheese and no milk. As a result life can be extremely difficult, and relatively few individuals who become vegetarians go this far. On a purely practical level, it is often impossible to obtain vegan food while travelling.

For the sake of completeness I should also point out that some vegans subsequently progress to fruitarianism — arguing that it is unethical to eat any living part of a plant, they try to exist entirely on a diet of fruit. There are a number of other equally rare variations on this rather extreme theme. Some individuals, who call themselves Hygienists, claim that cooked foods of any kind are bad for our health. They argue that raw foods are much better, and believe that it is vitally important for foods to be eaten in the correct pre-ordained combinations. There are also a few people who believe the opposite — that a diet containing fruit and raw vegetables is unhealthy. These individuals, who describe their dietary philosophy as Macrobiotics, aspire to a diet which consists of only brown rice.

Changing your diet is entirely a personal matter. You should never allow anyone whose eating habits are different from yours to make you feel guilty or irresponsible. Sadly, some vegetarians make it clear that they rather despise people who still eat fish or chicken, and some vegans do nothing to hide the fact that they haven't got much time for anyone who professes to be a vegetarian but who still enjoys a fried egg with their chips.

QUESTION: *What about meat substitutes? Are they really free of meat?*

ANSWER: *Yes, and some vegetarian hamburgers and sausages are pretty good – though others are absolutely terrible. I think meat-substitute products are all right occasionally, but I wouldn't recommend them as a regular part of your diet – they can get boring.*

Personally, I prefer to spend the money I save by not buying meat on trying out new foods. I recently discovered ugli fruit – half orange and half grapefruit. They're wonderful. And I'm not too keen on nut roasts – nuts are an excellent source of protein (though they are high in calories), but I prefer eating them whole to turning them into meat substitutes.

A few years ago I would have never thought that I would ever become any sort of vegetarian. Steak and kidney pie, bacon sandwiches and barbecued sausages were among my favourite meals. So I'm certainly not about to nail my shade of green to the mast and aver that I'll never give up eggs or cheese. But at the moment I feel comfortable with my dietary choice. And I certainly don't think that my decisions about my diet make me a better person than someone who eats steak twice a day or a worse person than someone who lives on a diet of brown rice.

All I know with any certainty is that today I feel comfortable about eating eggs and cheese but I don't feel comfortable about eating meat. Like many other vegetarians I went through a phase of eating white meat (mainly chicken) and no red meat, and then I went through a phase of eating fish but no meat. But eventually I decided that hauling fish out of their natural habitat so that I could smother them in vinegar and eat them with chips just wasn't something that I could justify.

QUESTION: *Is it safe for children to follow a vegetarian diet?*

ANSWER: *Yes – although I would have grave doubts about encouraging parents to bring up a child as a vegan. If a child has a balanced vegetarian diet which contains a healthy mixture of fresh foods, then he or she will get all the protein, vitamins and minerals that are needed. Most schools now provide meals or facilities for vegetarian children. A vegan diet, however, may be deficient in some essentials. If you want to bring up a child as a vegan make sure that you get expert advice from a nutritionist or dietician. Your GP should be able to put you in touch with someone local.*

I should perhaps point out that, although parents can bring up a child as a vegetarian, they should allow him or her to make a 'free' personal decision on the subject as adulthood approaches. It is never acceptable to try to force a moral code on anyone else. Having said that, I don't think it's any worse to encourage a healthy child to follow a vegetarian diet than it is to force a child to eat meat. The important thing is, I believe, to explain to the child why your diet does not include meat. If he or she becomes personally committed, then there will be no real problems at school or with friends.

I am satisfied that my brand of vegetarianism (a brand favoured by the vast majority of 'new' greens) allows me to eat without feeling guilt. I don't want to eat meat because I know that for me to have a chop on my plate an animal has to be killed. Further than that, by ensuring that I buy only free-range eggs and doing what I can to campaign for farm animals to be well looked after, I can help make sure that my eating habits don't mean that animals have to suffer. That is my moral argument for being a vegetarian rather than a vegan.

There are strong health arguments too. Because their diet contains no animal protein at all, vegans deprive themselves of several essential substances. Some amino acids aren't found in fruit or vegetables. Vitamin B12, which is needed for the formation of red blood cells, is also likely to be deficient. And vegans also run the risk of consuming too little iron, calcium, zinc and iodine. It is true that by taking great care many of these potential deficiencies can be dealt with. For example, there is iron in wholegrains, lentils and beans; zinc is found in wheatgerm, nuts and seeds; and it is possible to avert calcium deficiency by eating plenty of green leafy vegetables, wholefoods, nuts, pulses, seeds and soya milk. But there is no doubt that some vegans do suffer deficiency disorders, and many of them supplement their diet by swallowing pills.

Personally, I consider that any diet which requires supplementation with artificial pills prepared by the pharmaceutical industry (which has been responsible for a series of disgraceful abuses of humans) quite unacceptable. I am reluctant to choose a lifestyle which must inevitably lead to the boosting of their profits and the funding of their often quite indecent and cruel practices. I prefer to follow an entirely natural and wholesome diet.

QUESTION: *If I became a vegetaian do I have to stop wearing wool, leather and suede? I don't fancy the idea of wearing plastic sandals all the time.*

ANSWER: *My view is that the damage done to the environment by the manufacture of plastic clothes and shoes far exceeds any damage done by wearing the skins of animals which would have died anyway. I certainly would not buy any clothes made from material taken from an animal bred specifically for the purpose (for example fur coats). And I will not buy more shoes than I need simply so that I can look fashionable. But I do wear leather shoes and I do wear woollen jumpers. I realize that some strict vegans would regard this as unforgivable, but I regard their protests as hollow. After all, you could argue that the plastics industry – which manufactures many of the alternatives – has killed thousands of human beings as a serious polluter of the atmosphere and our rivers and seas. My advice is simple: you must do what you feel comfortable with (morally rather than physically!).*

Some vegans will undoubtedly claim that it is impossible to obtain eggs, milk or cheese without abusing animals. I disagree. I believe that it is perfectly possible to keep hens and cattle in comfortable conditions, and to obtain natural food products from them without cruelty or abuse.

I have, therefore, confined much of the advice in this book to those wishing to follow a largely vegetarian – rather than a vegan – diet. However, the recipe section (Chapter 9) does include a number of 'Dark Green' recipes suitable for vegans.

Is man a carnivore?

I don't think there are any neat black-and-white answers to this question. But it deserves an answer. No one is absolutely certain about what our early ancestors ate, but it seems pretty certain that most of them followed a non-specific diet – they were omnivorous. Primitive man ate what he could get – and although that probably included some meat, it almost certainly did not include regular quantities of it. There is little doubt that before animals such as the pig, cow and sheep were domesticated men would have had little chance of killing large wild animals with their primitive weapons. Would you fancy trying to catch a bison, a boar or a bear with only a small, slightly pointed rock? There does, however, seem to be some evidence that primitive man did eat small animals such as frogs and snails, and that they caught fish and crabs when they could.

On the whole, meat seems to have played a fairly small part in man's diet for many thousands of years until sophisticated weaponry and complex farming techniques made the killing of animals more feasible. When meat was available it was usually kept for religious ceremonies or for feasts with some traditional or cultural significance. The Australian Aboriginals seem fairly typical of primitive man – their usual diet consists largely of wild fruits and vegetables, supplemented with nuts, seeds, flowers, honey and occasional eggs. When they could catch animals they ate meat, but they didn't expect it as a regular part of their daily diet.

Certainly our physical structure seems to suggest that our basic, traditional diet was more herbivorous than carnivorous. For example, proper carnivores such as wolves, foxes, dogs and cats have large, powerful canine teeth and jaws which are suitable for biting and tearing animal flesh. Herbivores, on the other hand (such as cows and horses), have teeth and jaws which are designed for grinding and chewing vegetation. We do have canine teeth, but they are vestigial and not of much practical use. Compare the longest tooth in your mouth with the longest tooth in the mouth of your pet cat or dog, for example.

Our bowel structure also seems to support the theory that primitive man got most of his nourishment from plants rather than animals. Herbivores have long bowels so that they have time to extract essential nutrients from plants. Carnivores, who get their nutrients 'ready packed' in meat form, only need short bowels. The human bowel is long – in other words designed to extract as much nourishment as possible from a diet that is predominantly vegetarian.

The one thing which seems certain is that over the centuries our developing farming techniques have been responsible for many of the changes in our daily diet and food priorities. Over the years an industry has grown up to breed, feed and prepare for us a rich diet of fatty meat. In contrast the only meat our ancestors ever ate would have been lean and stringy. An animal caught in the wild contains a much lower fat content than one deliberately fattened in a stall in an artificially lit barn. Modern animals do no running about and get all the food they want. We do not have to use any physical effort to catch the meat we eat – we simply drive to the supermarket and pick out a joint of meat from the freezer.

While all these changes have taken place in farming and food preparation there have been relatively few changes to our bodies. It takes countless thousands or even millions of years for physiological characteristics to change. We have not managed to evolve as quickly as we have changed our world and our diet.

Our ancestors ate meat only occasionally: they drank blood to give themselves strength, and they ate the brains of their enemies in order to acquire their wisdom for themselves. Today, however, we have learned new eating habits. We have learned to regard meat as part of our regular, daily diet. We have learned to like the taste of fatty meat, and skilful marketing and advertising techniques mean that we readily accept meat as an apparently 'essential' part of our diet. We don't eat meat because we *have* to eat meat; we eat meat because we have been taught that we should eat meat.

In the last century or so our consumption of meat –

particularly fatty meat – has rocketed. For example, our consumption of battery-bred chickens is now some ten times higher than it was thirty-five years ago. Today a third or even a quarter of the unwanted fat in our diet comes from the meat we eat.

The true answer to the original question – whether man is a natural carnivore – is, I suspect, that he is an opportunist: he will eat whatever is available. He is, to some extent, a scavenger. Our closest relatives – the gorillas – never eat meat, and most other members of the monkey family eat very little of it. But man has been blessed with mental and physical skills which have enabled him to 'farm' other animals, to create new breeds of domesticated animals which can be bred specially for food.

Over the years we have become accustomed to having meat in our diet. In the past it was regarded as something of a luxury; today it is thought of as an essential. We have allowed the farmers and their advertising and marketing experts to persuade us to eat enormous quantities of poor-quality meat. Today many people have difficulty in planning a meal without meat as its focal point. There are many other useful sources of protein, but meat is regarded as the 'king' of foods. Baked beans on wholemeal toast is without doubt one of the healthiest meals in the world, but many people would consider the meanest and cheapest meat product to be superior.

The final, unavoidable truth is that it is man's ability to think creatively which has enabled him to domesticate animals for his own consumption. And yet it seems to me that our modern, newly established tradition of abusing animals to make them a regular part of our diet reflects the dark side of our nature. We have been blessed with the capacity for thought, and this blessing means that we surely cannot continue to allow our darkest nature to rule our behaviour.

Human beings were probably designed to eat a mixed diet. A million or so years ago our ancestors ate whatever they could get their hands on. Most of the time they lived on plants and plant products. Only occasionally did they get the chance to add meat to their diet. It was only when our ancestors learned to control fire, a modest half a million years ago, that they were able to start cooking meat and making it more digestible.

The truth of the matter is that, although we may be designed in such a way that we can eat meat, we were never designed to eat as much meat as we've become accustomed to consuming. And we were certainly never built to cope with a diet full of fat-rich meat.

The animals our ancestors caught were lean and rather stringy. Thousands of years of commercial farming have turned once wild animals into completely different beasts. The simple truth is that you and I were never designed to eat a fatted calf.

The facts about your food

In an average lifetime of seventy years each one of us eats around thirty tons of food. The food we eat supplies the materials we need in order to grow and to repair and rebuild damaged tissues. Proteins from that food supply the amino acids with which our bodies build up all the essential human body proteins. Vitamins and minerals are used, alongside enzymes, to help operate metabolic processes inside the body.

In addition to providing essential nutrients for building, repairing and operating our bodies, the food we eat also provides us with the energy we need to keep our bodies warm, to keep our organs operating and to enable us to use our muscles. The more exercise we do, the more food we need.

If we consume more food than our bodies need for everyday work, the residue is converted into body fat. If at some time in the future our food intake falls below our body's needs, then the stored fat will be brought into use and converted into energy.

The food we eat is made up of carbohydrates, fats, proteins, vitamins and minerals. Following is a description of the different roles and characteristics of these various ingredients.

Carbohydrates

What a terrible reputation carbohydrates have among slimmers! And yet, surprisingly perhaps, most people in developed countries – and most slimmers – take too little of their daily food intake in the form of carbohydrates.

Carbohydrates are manufactured by plants – vegetables, fruits and cereals – using water, sunlight and the waste gas breathed out by human beings, carbon dioxide. There are three basic types of plant carbohydrates: fibre or roughage, sugars or simple carbohydrates, and starches or complex carbohydrates.

Fibre has been extremely fashionable for several years now, and a number of companies have made a great deal of money out of packaging and selling it as though it was some newly discovered, magical ingredient. The truth is, however, that the explosion in the demand for fibre has been created by the discovery of the fact that for years now food manufacturers have been taking far too much of it out of our natural foodstuffs. Undoubtedly they thought they were doing us all a terrific favour: fibre doesn't contain very much of any obvious nutritional significance, and most of it goes straight through our intestinal tracts more or less unchanged.

But what the food refiners didn't realize is that, although it may not appear to be of any great nutritional significance, fibre is an extremely important part of our daily diet. Over several million years our digestive systems have been developed to deal with food which contains fibre. It is the fibre in the food you eat which gives your bowels something to squeeze. Fibre helps to stimulate the whole digestive system, helps to keep food moving and helps to prevent problems such as constipation.

QUESTION: *Will becoming a vegetarian have any good effects on my health?*

ANSWER: *It could have. If you suffer from constipation, for example, you'll probably find that eating more fresh fruit and vegetables will solve your problem permanently. The extra fibre in plant food will help enormously. You will also be far less likely to suffer from food poisoning – over 90 per cent of food poisoning cases are due to infected meat. You'll find a fairly extensive account of the advantages of a low-meat or meat-free diet in later parts of this book.*

A few years ago doctors noticed that certain diseases which

were becoming increasingly common in America and Europe were almost unknown in the less well-developed countries, where eating habits were still relatively primitive and where processed white bread was unheard of. Slowly the medical profession managed to demonstrate that people who eat a diet which is too low in fibre run the risk of developing a wide range of digestive problems. They also proved that since fibre fills us up, and provides few calories and helps to reduce the absorption of fat and slow down the absorption of sugar, it is of enormous importance to slimmers.

Although food processing plants have changed a great deal in the last few decades, our intestines haven't altered at all. Our bodies still need a good, regular supply of roughage. The list of diseases now known to be associated with a low-fibre diet includes: bowel cancer, diverticular disease of the bowel (a muscle abnormality which results in the development of small pockets in the bowel wall), appendicitis, gallstones and varicose veins. As a general rule most of us need to eat considerably more fibre. On average we need to eat more or less double our normal daily intake of it if we are to eat a healthier diet and avoid that long list of disorders just mentioned.

But although we need more fibre we don't need to start buying special fibre or bran supplements. It is much better to get the extra roughage we need from natural foodstuffs. It is also much cheaper! I find it remarkable that food companies which have taken the fibre out of the food they sell us then have the nerve to offer us the fibre back again as a high-cost supplement! This must surely be one of the great confidence tricks of all time.

Fibre comes from plant cell walls and is made up of a number of complex carbohydrates. There are two main types of fibre: soluble fibre and insoluble fibre. Most foods which contain fibre include both types.

The richest sources of soluble fibre are pulses – peas and beans – and products such as porridge, pearl barley or rye bread that contain oats, barley or rye. However, most vegetables and fruits contain some soluble fibre.

Once you've eaten soluble fibre it forms a sticky, jelly-like substance in your stomach and restricts the amount of fat you

Fibre

You should increase your intake of fibre because:
- it will help you feel full – and reduce your appetite
- it will reduce the risk of suffering from stomach and bowel problems
- it will reduce the risk of suffering from gallstones, varicose veins and appendicitis
- it will help reduce the amount of fat your body absorbs
- it will help you avoid constipation
- it will help absorb toxins and poisons – and prevent them being absorbed into your body
- fibre-rich food needs more chewing – and is, therefore, better prepared for digestion when it reaches your stomach

To increase your intake of fibre:
- eat more bread – preferably wholemeal; cut it thick
- eat more pasta – especially wholewheat
- eat more rice – particularly brown
- use wholewheat or wholemeal flour when cooking
- eat oats (in porridge) and bran-rich cereals
- eat more fresh vegetables and fruit
- eat dried fruits and nuts instead of chocolate and sweets
- eat more pulses (e.g. baked beans)
- when buying biscuits choose wholemeal oat ones
- eat potatoes in jackets
- add shredded or grated raw vegetables to salads
- make biscuits and crumbles with rolled oats
- do not peel fruit or vegetables, but do wash well first
- don't cook vegetables for long – and cook in as little water as possible.

Note: Increase your intake of fibre gradually. Many people suffer from wind and abdominal discomfort if they eat too much fibre too quickly.

can absorb from the food you've eaten. It is also soluble fibre which slows down the rate at which sugar is absorbed into the body. Additionally, by helping to control the production of insulin (the hormone which controls blood sugar levels) soluble fibre probably helps to stop you feeling hungry.

In contrast insoluble fibre is found mainly in vegetables such as spring greens and in products such as flour, bread and breakfast cereals which are made from wheat. Insoluble fibre acts more like a sponge than a jelly and swells as it soaks up the moisture in our stomachs. It is because it swells up that insoluble fibre makes us feel full and stops us eating too much.

The second type of carbohydrate is sugar. The sugars we use most commonly are the refined white or brown varieties sold in bags in the supermarket. These types of sugar are also known as sucrose, and they are produced from either sugar cane or sugar beet. They are rich in calories but contain virtually no other useful nutrients, so they provide instant energy but little else. There are, however, many other types of sugar – including honey, treacle, blackstrap molasses, corn syrup, glucose, fructose and maltose.

Some of these other types of sugar do include additional useful ingredients. For example, honey contains a few vitamins and minerals, while blackstrap molasses has a little calcium and iron as well as other minerals. But these differences are slight and, despite the extravagant claims made by some health food shops, there are really no reasons to eat honey or other substances in preference to ordinary sugar. Nor is it at all true that honey made by bees which have collected particular types of pollen has any special value.

Today food manufacturers add sugar to just about everything from soup (to bring out the flavour and 'improve' the texture) to tinned meat (to keep the product 'soft') to tomato sauce (to make it smoother) to biscuits (to make them crunchy and crumbly). By ensuring that most refined and packaged foods contain a hefty dose of sugar, by promoting sugar as an essential foodstuff and by spreading a false message that sugar is harmless, the food manufacturers ensure that on average each one of us consumes nearly 100lb (45kg) of sugar a year. There are, however, a number of problems associated with eating too much sugar. Independent researchers have shown a strong association with tooth decay and with cancers of the breast, colon and rectum. In addition there is no doubt that the

Sugar

You should reduce your intake of sugar because:
- it will cause tooth decay
- it will make you fat
- it will increase your risk of developing heart disease and other serious problems
- large quantities of sugar increase your risk of developing cancer of the breast, colon and rectum

To reduce your intake of sugar:
- read the labels on packaged foods and avoid buying products that contain added sugar
- eat dried fruits and nuts instead of sweets
- gradually reduce the amount of sugar used in tea or coffee – alternatively try drinking fewer cups of tea and coffee, or use artificial sweeteners
- choose low-calorie drinks or mineral water instead of sugar-rich soft drinks
- buy natural fruit juices instead of the sweetened varieties
- don't buy baby foods that contain added sugar
- don't add unnecessary sugar to milk when feeding a baby
- when baking add less sugar than recipes suggest – try cutting down a little more each time
- buy low-sugar jams and marmalades
- choose low-sugar biscuits (instead of biscuits coated with chocolate or filled with cream)
- eat fresh fruit rather than tinned – if you buy tinned fruit, go for products in juice rather than sugar-rich syrup
- buy natural unsweetened yoghurt – and add your own fruit for flavouring
- make puddings with less sugar
- when cooking, use other flavours, e.g. spices or fruits, instead of sugar
- when eating out, choose a low-fat cheese or fresh fruit instead of a high-sugar, high-fat pudding
- spread jam and marmalade more thinly on bread and toast

consumption of large quantities of sugar leads to obesity, which leads in turn to heart disease and a lot of other problems.

Incidentally, although some sugars – such as fructose, glucose and lactose – are found naturally in foods such as fruit, there is little doubt that refined or extracted sugars are far more likely to cause problems than sugars in their natural state, where they are mixed with plenty of fibre.

The third and final group of carbohydrates are the starches or 'complex carbohydrates'. Unlike simple sugars which are broken down quickly – and can be turned into 'instant' energy – the starches are usually digested slowly.

Starches

You should increase your intake of starches because:
- foods that are rich in starchy carbohydrates also contain protein, iron and vitamins
- starchy carbohydrates contain relatively few calories
- starchy carbohydrates are also rich in fibre

To increase your intake of starches:
- eat more bread, and cut it more thickly
- eat more vegetables
- eat more fresh fruit
- eat more rice
- eat more pasta
- eat more pulses – beans and peas

Foods such as pulses (peas and beans), cereals, rice, pasta and many different fruits and vegetables are rich in starches. It is clear, therefore, that a vegetarian – who inevitably eats many green vegetables, a lot of different fresh fruit and, often a considerable amount of bread, pasta and rice – must consume a lot of starch. Slimmers who find this worrying (since they associate carbohydrates with calories) should relax. Starchy carbohydrate foods do contain a good deal of potential energy (essential for daily life), but they also contain a wide range of other essential nutrients such as proteins, vitamins and minerals. Contrary to what slimmers frequently think, starchy carbohydrates are relatively low in calories and do not need to be avoided by people who want to get – and stay – slim.

QUESTION: *If I stop eating meat won't I become weak and easily tired?*

ANSWER: *No. Vegetarians have won Olympic medals in strength and endurance events. There have been vegetarian boxing champions. Some of the world's strongest animals – elephants, gorillas, bulls and horses – are vegetarian. By and large vegetarians are stronger and have more endurance – than meat-eaters.*

Fats

Your body gets much of its energy from the fat you eat. Unwanted supplies of energy are then stored as fat in all the old familiar places around your body. *Some* fat is an essential part of your diet, but unfortunately most of us eat far too much of it. On average half our calorie intake is delivered from the fat we eat, most of which comes from meat, meat products and dairy products such as milk, butter and cream. I doubt if there is any aspect of nutrition that causes more controversy and confusion than the subject of fats. So here are the answers to the questions people most commonly ask.

What is the difference between saturated, unsaturated and polyunsaturated fats?

All types of fat contain the same number of calories – and are equally fattening. All fats are also made up of the same basic types of fatty acids: saturated, unsaturated and polyunsaturated. The difference lies in the proportion of saturated to polyunsaturated fatty acids, and the three names are usually applied to fats according to the type of fatty acid that predominates.

It is saturated fats which cause most trouble. They commonly come from animals, in the form of meat or dairy products. Because we can't digest saturated fats properly they tend to stay in our bloodstream for long periods. Eventually they cling to the inner linings of our blood vessels, producing atherosclerosis, a narrowing that can eventually lead to high blood pressure, heart disease and strokes. The presence of large quantities of saturated fats also stops us metabolizing food properly – as well as preventing the removal of waste products. In the end diseases as varied as gout and diabetes can be caused by eating too much saturated fat.

You can tell how rich a fat is in saturated fatty acids by looking at it. Those fats which contain large quantities of saturated fatty acids are usually hard at room temperature – like lard and butter. The less saturated or unsaturated ones are mostly liquid fats or oils and are usually found in vegetable or plant oils, some of which, such as sunflower oil and safflower oil, are high in polyunsaturated fatty acids.

Just to add to the confusion there are some exceptions to these general rules. Palm oil and coconut oil – both plant oils which you might expect to be low in saturated fat — are, in fact, very high in saturated fat; while chicken, turkey, rabbit and oily fish such as mackerel, herrings and tuna contain less saturated fat than beef or pork.

What is cholesterol?

Cholesterol isn't the same thing as fat; although it has some similar properties, it is chemically known as a sterol and is present in all animal tissues. In moderation cholesterol isn't harmful, but if the level of cholesterol in your blood reaches too high a concentration then it can cause trouble – many experts now believe that the higher your blood cholesterol level, the greater the risk of your having a heart attack.

Although cholesterol is present in many of the things we eat, that isn't the *only* way that we can accumulate too much of the stuff: our bodies make their own cholesterol from saturated fats, so if you consume too many of them then your blood cholesterol level will almost certainly rise. Unsaturated fats, on the other hand, while they have the same energy level as saturated fats, tend to reduce blood cholesterol levels.

If you want to cut down your blood cholesterol levels you can do so in two ways. First, cut down your consumption of foods which themselves contain cholesterol – that means brains, caviar, cheese, chocolate, cream, eggs, heart, kidneys, liver, shellfish like crab and lobster, and sweetbreads. You don't have to cut out these foods completely – just cutting down will usually help. Second, cut down your consumption of animal fats such as butter, full cream milk, cooking fat and meat fat, which are rich in saturated fatty acids. All those fats can be turned into cholesterol once they get into your body. Remember, too, that palm oil and coconut oil are both rich in saturated fatty acids and are therefore also likely to lead to cholesterol problems.

Is fat bad for you?

It is essential to have some fat in your diet if you're going to stay healthy. Some polyunsaturated fatty acids, known as 'essential fatty acids or EFAs', are needed for the maintenance of cell membranes and for the production of substances such as prostaglandins which have a host of vital functions. But all the evidence now suggests that you should try to keep your consumption of saturated fats to a minimum. If you eat unlimited animal fats, then you will run a higher-than-average risk of developing arterial disease and having a heart attack.

The first likely connection between fat intake and heart disease was recorded back in 1953. Since then there have been

---

Fats

You should reduce your intake of saturated fat because:
- saturated fat will increase your risk of developing heart disease, high blood pressure and strokes
- saturated fat is rich in calories
- too much saturated fat will increase your blood cholesterol level
- high levels of saturated fat will clog up your arteries and reduce the efficiency of your blood

---

To reduce your intake of fats you should:

- drink skimmed or semi-skimmed milk
- buy better-tasting bread – and use less butter
- instead of butter use a low-fat spread or one which is high in polyunsaturates – remember that ordinary margarine contains saturated fats
- eat low-fat yoghurt and low-fat cheese
- if you must buy cream, buy single rather than double
- buy low-fat salad dressings, sausages and cakes
- buy lean meat – and cut off all visible fat
- eat more white meat, e.g. chicken
- eat more fish
- cook in oil that contains polyunsaturates
- grill rather than fry food
- drain off fat after cooking
- don't add fat when cooking
- make low-fat pastry
- don't eat the skin on chicken – it's high in fat
- cut chips more thickly – they soak up less fat than thin ones
- make sure the fat or oil is sizzling hot before you add chips – they will soak up less fat
- use herbs rather than fatty, oily salad dressings
- use herbs rather than butter on vegetables
- replace cream in recipes with yoghurt
- use the microwave if you have one – it means you don't have to add fat before cooking food
- use a non-stick pan when you fry – it means you don't have to add fat
- grill, bake, steam, poach, casserole and boil rather than roast or fry; stir-frying uses little fat
- dry chips on kitchen paper after cooking to remove any excess oil
- use oil in baking instead of hard fats
- after grilling or cooking meat on a rack (so that the fat drips out) throw the fat away rather than try to find a use for it

many more links added to the chain of evidence. In America, between 1963 and 1975 the consumption of milk, butter and other animal fats went down dramatically. During the same period the heart attack rate also fell noticeably.

More startling evidence has come from Belgium. For twenty years the Flemish-speaking people living in the north of the country have been steadily reducing the amount of fat they eat. In the south, however, the French-speaking population kept its consumption of fat fairly high. By early 1970 the average northener was eating only 80 per cent of the fat that was being consumed by the average southerner.

It is difficult to avoid the conclusion that there is a strong link between the amount of fat eaten and the incidence of heart disease. Just about every major scientific and medical committee in the world now agrees that saturated fats cause heart disease. And just about every expert in the world agrees that we would all be wise to cut down our consumption of fat – especially saturated fat. In America a special Senate committee set up to study health and diet recommended that the consumption of fats be cut from 40 per cent of the average energy intake to 30 per cent.

QUESTION: *Do vegetarians live longer?*

ANSWER: *Most vegetarians are probably healthier than most meat-eaters. But that is probably because vegetarians tend to be more conscious of their health than meat-eaters. As a group they smoke less and probably take more exercise. Because meat (and meat products) are rich in fat anyone who cuts down on his or her meat consumption will be less prone to disorders such as heart disease, which are known to be associated with a high fat intake. Giving up meat and fish completely will not, however, improve your life expectation.*

Of course, all this has not gone unchallenged – particularly by those who have a vested financial interest in maintaining the sales of fat (and especially of animal products) at a high level. Those who dispute the evidence linking a high-fat diet to the incidence of heart disease do not, however, have the luxury of vast quantities of scientific evidence with which to support their argument. Instead, certain pressure groups have used what some might view as slightly underhand techniques to try to maintain their market share.

In most countries, confusion about the danger of fat has been maintained by a number of paid pressure groups. Every year thousands of men and women die prematurely in their thirties and forties because they have been encouraged to eat unlimited quantities of fat. The credit for this must go to the farmers and food manufacturers, who between them have organized a powerful lobby to disguise and distort the truth about animal fats. Since they have an obvious commercial interest in ensuring that we all continue to eat lots of butter, eggs and fatty meat, and to wash it all down with lots of full cream milk, farmers and food manufacturers have joined forces to fund a number of extremely effective and ruthless propaganda organizations.

They pay out huge sums on advertising, but they also use their spending power to try and influence public opinion in more subtle ways. For example, after I appeared on one British TV station and told viewers that a high-fat diet containing too much butter and milk could lead to heart disease, the station boss received a letter from an executive of the Butter Information Council. The writer pointed out that his organization had been about to spend a large sum of money on TV advertising, and that this plan had 'come under review' as a result of my remarks.

The unavoidable truth, however, is that too much fat *is* bad for you. Saturated fat won't just clog up your blood vessels; it will also reduce the efficiency with which your red blood cells carry oxygen around your body, and it will pick up and accumulate waste products which should be excreted.

Cutting down your total fat intake will cut down your calorie intake. Cutting down your saturated fat intake will improve your health.

Protein

We make our own body proteins from the amino acids we obtain from the proteins we eat. And protein is essential for the body's growth, for tissue repair and for food metabolism. Its constituents are long chains of amino acids, of which there are twenty-two types in the human body. All amino acids contain nitrogen. Eight of the amino acids which are used to create adult proteins, and ten of the amino acids used to create

QUESTION: *How do you explain the fact that my grandfather lived to be ninety-four even though he ate meat and animal fats all his life?*

ANSWER: *Statistically, one case history is totally meaningless. I know a man who has been involved in three separate car crashes. That doesn't mean that car crashes are good for you – or even that they are harmless. I know several heavy smokers who have celebrated their seventieth birthdays, but that doesn't mean that thousands of other individuals haven't died in their thirties or forties because they've smoked. To draw any useful conclusions about diet and health you need to study large groups of people. When you do so it becomes clear that there is a strong link between the consumption of large quantities of animal fat and the development of disorders such as strokes, high blood pressure and heart disease.*

There are three other reasons why your grandfather might have lived to ninety-four on a diet rich in fat. First, there is little doubt that the amount of fat in meat has changed fairly dramatically over the last twenty or thirty years. Today cattle farmers deliberately fatten up their animals so that they will get more money for them. There are even some bizarre regulations which mean that animals have to contain a certain amount of fat before they are killed. A few decades ago animals were leaner and eating their meat was less hazardous to your health.

Second, your grandfather probably ate far more fibre than most modern meat-eaters. Half a century ago refined, packaged foodstuffs were used much less widely. Vegetables were eaten fresh, and bread full of roughage was eaten in fairly large quantities.

Third, your grandfather's lifestyle was most probably different from yours. Earlier this century people took far more exercise than they do today. There were fewer motor cars around, and travelling somewhere usually meant walking at least part of the way. In addition there were fewer other machines available: most heavy work had to be done by hand. To all this you must add the fact that the degree of stress in people's lives was considerably less half or a quarter of a century ago. Today most of us have too much stress in our lives – and do too little natural exercise; we desperately need a healthy diet in order to cope with the world we have created for ourselves.

proteins in children, have to be obtained in the food we eat because our bodies cannot make them. These are known as 'essential' amino acids.

Protein

You should eat a balanced supply of protein because:

- it is essential for growth and for the repair of damaged tissues; it is also essential for the production of some enzymes
- if you eat too little protein then tissue proteins – particularly muscles – will be broken down
- if you eat more protein than is necessary the constituent amino acids will be broken down and some of the protein converted into body fat. Eating too much protein may also increase the loss of calcium from your body – with an increased risk of osteoporosis developing. In addition too much protein may put a strain on your liver and kidneys (because large amounts of amino acids have to be broken down and the nitrogen excreted). Scientists have also suggested that people who eat a high-protein diet (this usually means one that contains too much meat) run a risk of developing vitamin deficiency. It has also been suggested that a high-protein diet may lead to cancers (particularly breast cancer) and heart disease. Japanese women living in their own country run a low risk of developing breast cancer, but those living in America and eating approximately four times as much meat are far more likely to develop this disease.

In the past, foods which contained adequate quantities of the essential amino acids were called 'first-class proteins'. Most of these 'first-class proteins' came from meat and other animal products. Foods which did not contain adequate quantities of the 'essential' amino acids were known as 'second-class proteins'. Most of these came from plant foods.

QUESTION: *Is a vegetarian diet deficient in any essential proteins or vitamins? If I stop eating meat won't I need to take special supplements in order to stay healthy?*

ANSWER: *The short, simple answer to both questions is 'No'. It is quite true that most of us get the majority of our protein from meat – but that is purely because of our eating habits. For a variety of cultural, social and commercial reasons we tend to eat meat or fish at most main meals. But the fact is that meat is certainly not the only potential source of protein. Animal products are, pound for pound, only a very slightly better source of protein than nuts or seeds and no better than things like soya beans. You can get all the protein you need from a vegetarian diet.*

The same is true of vitamins and minerals. It is a myth that meat contains essential vitamins and minerals that can't be obtained any other way. Although vegans may need to take supplements, vegetarians who still eat eggs and dairy products (and who take care to eat a good, balanced diet) will be able to get all the vitamins and minerals they need.

Although this type of classification is still used by some older nutritionists, it is rather out-of-date now. Today it is recognized that just about any good balanced diet will include all the amino acids needed to create new proteins. You may also hear some so-called experts refer to 'complete' and 'incomplete' proteins when talking about amino acids. I suggest that you ignore such nonsense. Anyone who talks about 'complete' and 'incomplete' proteins or 'first-class' or 'second-class' proteins is showing himself or herself to be woefully out of touch with reality. You can get all the amino acids your body needs in order to manufacture its protein supplies without eating any meat or meat products at all – vegans get an adequate supply just from the plants they eat.

Some bizarre individuals also claim that in order to satisfy your body's amino acid requirements you must eat specific types of protein together – so that the right amino acids get into your body in the right order. This shows a rather charming naivety, suggesting that the human body is so simple and inefficient that it cannot possibly look after itself if the ingredients for survival are not provided in absolutely the right order. It is rather like saying that your pocket calculator won't be able to add up figures properly if you don't key in the separate parts of your sum in a pre-ordained sequence.

Despite the lack of scientific logic behind it, however, 'food combining' does seem to have attracted a lot of support. Some journalists (most of the people advocating this theory have no medical or scientific qualifications whatsoever) claim that you should only ever eat cheese with bread; others claim that you will do your body permanent damage if you eat fruit with meat; and many seem to believe that eating potatoes in the wrong order is likely to lead to physical ruination.

There is some truth in the suggestion that you should try to eat a balanced diet – with each meal made up of different types of food – but I really don't think you need be concerned about the order in which each forkful goes into your mouth! As long as you eat a good and varied diet your body can sort things out for itself very nicely, thank you.

It is also true that, although animal produce is traditionally the primary source of protein, for most of us it is, gram for gram, only a marginally better source of protein than nuts and seeds and no better than soya beans. Once inside your body proteins – whether they come in the form of meat or plant – are broken down into their component parts. The various amino acids are then absorbed into your body and used to make the proteins and enzymes that your body needs to stay alive. By and large the younger you are the better your body will be at making new protein – so the quicker wounds will heal and the more you'll grow. Because they are growing rapidly, children need more protein than adults do.

The human body can't store protein in the same way that it can store fat, and so you have to eat more or less what you need fairly regularly. The difference between the amount of nitrogen you take in – in the form of amino acids – and the amount your body excretes as waste is known as your nitrogen balance. When your body is growing or repairing damaged tissues you will keep far more nitrogen than you excrete; while if you are not eating enough and your body has to break down body proteins in order to provide you with energy, then you will excrete more nitrogen than you are taking in. The first of these two conditions is described as having a positive nitrogen balance; the second is known as a negative nitrogen balance. Normally, your body will be in balance – with equal quantities of nitrogen coming in and going out.

Vitamins and minerals

Sometimes called 'micro-nutrients', because we need them in such minute quantities, vitamins and minerals are essential for our bodies to stay alive. They help keep our body tissues and skin healthy; produce enzymes to help in a whole range of essential activities; aid the release of energy from the food we eat; help keep nerves in good condition; and assist in the production of hormones and red blood cells. Without vitamins and minerals our teeth and bones would crumble and we would die.

When vitamins were first discovered half a century ago they were given letters as they were identified – A, B, C, D and so on. Then scientists discovered that the substance they had called vitamin B actually consisted of several *different* substances, so they began to rename the vitamins in the B group, calling them B1, B2, B3, B4 and so on. Just to add to the confusion many vitamins – particularly those in the B group – are also given names; for example, vitamin B1 is known as thiamine and sometimes aneurin, and B2 as riboflavin. The most important vitamins are undoubtedly vitamins A, B group, C and D.

Many people who give up eating meat, or just cut down, worry that their diet will not contain enough vitamins and minerals. This well-established fear has been largely nurtured by journalists who have failed to do their research properly. The fact is that it really isn't easy to become vitamin-deficient. For example, devising a diet which does not contain enough vitamin E is almost impossible. Similarly, it is fairly difficult to run short of supplies of other vitamins. Even wartime concentration camp inmates, desperately short of food, often turned out to have a reasonably satisfactory intake of vitamins.

There is vitamin A in milk, eggs, butter, cheese, liver and fish oils. However, if you are a vegetarian you can get your supplies from vegetables which contain a substance called carotene.

Vitamin B is found in a wide range of foods, which include both animal and vegetable products. A shortage of vitamin B1 can result in a very unpleasant disease known as beri-beri, but you'll be safe enough from this if your diet includes cereals. Even refined flour has vitamins added to make up for what has been lost in the polishing. The best-known vitamin problem associated with vegetarianism involves vitamin B12, which does come mainly from meat, fish and dairy food. Without enough B12 we develop pernicious anaemia — though the human liver can store B12 for two or three years. You can, however, obtain enough B12 if you eat some dairy produce; and even vegans, who eat no animal products at all, can avoid a deficiency if they take great care with their diet (see page 48).

Getting enough vitamin C is absolutely no problem for vegetarians, because most fruit and vegetables contain the vitamin in large quantities. Indeed, meat-eaters are more likely to suffer from scurvy — the classic disease associated with vitamin C deficiency — than are vegetarians.

Vitamin D is no problem either. The human body can make its own vitamin D with the aid of a little sunshine, and there are very few countries in the world where the supply of sunshine is inadequate. The only vegetarians at risk of developing vitamin D deficiency are those who are dark-skinned — their skin may be less capable of making vitamin D in countries where the sunshine is weak. This need not be a major difficulty, however, since vitamin D is present in many foodstuffs — there is, for example, lots of it in dairy foods.

As long as you eat a balanced diet there is little risk of you developing any real vitamin deficiency. The same thing is true for minerals. The one mineral that vegetarians worry most about is iron. But dark green vegetables, peas, beans and dried fruit all contain it. Indeed, meat-eaters are often more likely to suffer from iron deficiency than are vegetarians, since the absorption of iron into the body is achieved far more efficiently when the diet contains a reasonable amount of vitamin C.

If you follow the eating advice in this book you are unlikely to suffer from any vitamin or mineral deficiency. All the available evidence shows that the people who are most at risk are the ones who eat too much processed, heavily refined food and too little natural food. Going on crash diets and eating food out of packets and tins is far more likely to lead to nutritional deficiencies than following a vegetarian diet.

And don't worry too much about trying to ensure that your *daily* intake of food contains all the various minerals and vitamins you need – the human body is very good at storing small quantities of most of the essential supplies it needs. The important thing is to make sure that you balance your diet on a long-term basis.

Are vitamin and mineral supplements helpful?

The short answer to this question has to be an emphatic 'No!' I believe that the vitamin business is currently one of the biggest cons in the world. Every week millions of otherwise intelligent and well-informed individuals spend a small fortune on vitamin and mineral supplements. The market for these pills has grown steadily for years now, and the shelves of your local health food shop and pharmacy will undoubtedly be groaning under their weight. Once the companies selling these products have recruited a new customer they can usually rely on him (or her) remaining faithful for life. Many customers develop a psychological addiction to their tablets — they believe that they are going to feel better when they take them, and so they *do* feel better. Once that has happened it is nigh on impossible for them to stop.

The manufacture and sale of vitamin supplements is nothing new, of course. Back in 1923 the editors of the *British Medical Journal* were so worried about what they saw as a new and unnecessary phenomenon that they published an article entitled 'The vitamin content of certain proprietary preparations', written by a team including the then Professor of Pharmacology at the University of London. The conclusion of the authors was that:

our experiments confirm that what other workers on vitamins have emphasised – namely that under normal conditions of life an adequate supply of vitamins can easily be ensured by including in the diet a suitable amount of protective foods such as milk, butter, green vegetables and fruit and that no advantage is to be gained by trying to obtain the substances in the form of drugs.

That was fifty years ago, but the companies selling vitamins have continued to promote their products with all sorts of pseudo-scientific arguments, creating and then satisfying a series of quite artificial needs. One of the most successful marketing strategies was to announce that vitamin C could be used to help fight off colds. This suggestion was discredited back in the mid-1970s by a series of comprehensive trials which showed quite conclusively that there was no scientific basis to the claim. In one of the most damning pieces of evidence, published in the *Journal of the American Medical Association*, details were given of a trial in which a number of Marine recruits were each given 2 gram doses of vitamin C in an attempt to stop them getting colds (2 grams is an enormous dose). The researchers were able to show that the pills had no protective effect whatsoever.

But all the research has still not managed to destroy this vitamin's reputation as a cure-all, and there are many people who continue to take their daily vitamin C pills in the belief that they are reducing their risk of catching colds. The truth, as proved in numerous scientific experiments, is that vitamin C supplements will only help provide you with some protection if your body is short of this vitamin (in other words, if you are suffering from scurvy) and if your diet is also deficient in it. Since vitamin C is water-soluble and cannot be stored in the human body in any sizeable quantities, the excess taken by people whose diets include lots of fruit and vegetables and other vitamin C-rich foods is simply excreted in the urine.

Maybe because they recognize that the sale of vitamin supplements cannot continue unabated forever, a number of companies are now selling a large range of mineral supplements too. One of the most fashionable and commercially successful of these is zinc, and thousands of innocent consumers are already taking extra zinc in the hope that their brainpower and sex lives will be boosted. Many people who can ill afford these unnecessary extras are buying them because they believe that they are essential for good health.

One press hand-out I have seen contained the assertion that zinc is linked to virtually every aspect of human growth, development and wellbeing. It has been colourfully and inaccurately described as 'penicillin for the mind', and at least forty different conditions – including anorexia, depression, delayed sexual maturation and low birth weight – have been blamed on zinc deficiency. Unfortunately, a little investigation shows that these claims are over-optimistic and potentially misleading. Another press release states that 'adequate supplementation will probably reduce the risk of contracting most diseases, from the acute common cold to common infections', but the world's medical journals are light on supporting evidence.

These advertising assertions seem to me to be based on no more than theory, enthusiasm and anecdotes – with a few rather optimistic conclusions thrown in for good measure. For example, one of the pieces of evidence usually produced to support the contention that zinc supplements are useful in the treatment of anorexia is a report published in the *Lancet* in 1984. But this report dealt with just one patient, and was greeted by specialists with some scepticism. An expert on anorexia said there was not a spot of serious evidence that the cure worked; even a leading expert on zinc shared that doubt. I was similarly unimpressed when I examined the rest of the evidence cited to support the claims made for zinc.

As a second example, consider germanium. I have in front of me a book which suggests that germanium can be used in the treatment of the following conditions:

angina	glaucoma
arthritis	heart attack
asthma	herpes
breast cancer	high blood pressure
burns	influenza
cancer of the colon	leukaemia
cancer of the prostate	lung cancer
cataracts	malaria
cervical cancer	osteoporosis
corns	ovarian cancer
depression	Parkinson's disease
detached retina	rheumatism
diabetes	schizophrenia
eczema	stomach and duodenal ulcers
epilepsy	stroke
gastritis	warts

To me all this seems frighteningly irresponsible. Germanium is a trace element which used to play a part in the manufacture of transistors for radios. I have been unable to find any convincing evidence that germanium supplements can be used to treat this wide range of disorders. In my view an ordinary, well-balanced diet will contain all the germanium anyone needs. Furthermore, I believe that extra supplements are more likley to do harm than to do good; I have already read a report suggesting that one man died of kidney failure after taking germanium supplements.

It is, I think, perhaps worth pointing out that the profits to be made from these products are enormous. Zinc, for example, is exceedingly cheap. For the over-the-counter price of a month's supply for one person, the supplement manufacturer can buy enough to supply a small town.

The plain, unvarnished, uncommercial truth is that if you eat sensibly you will automatically get enough vitamins and minerals in your diet. If you don't eat sensibly it won't just be extra vitamins that you need – and the supplements you require should be prescribed by a doctor, who can carry out the necessary blood tests and then prescribe exactly what you need in the correct quantities. Eating extra vitamins to get healthy or stay fitter is about as logical as trying to pump an extra thousand gallons of petrol into your car in the hope that it will go faster, or attempting to pump another million volts into your TV set to get a better picture.

As a final thought, I do not know of a single doctor who takes vitamin or mineral supplements. If taking vitamin and mineral supplements was good for your health, then presumably the medical profession would have caught on and would be among the keenest of all pill poppers. They aren't, and they haven't.

Can you take too many vitamins or minerals?

There is no doubt at all about this – the answer is an unequivocal 'Yes!' Most vitamin and mineral manufacturers and advocates fail to tell their customers that supplements can be dangerous, but since supplements became popular the dangers have been well documented and there is now an overwhelming body of evidence. Too many vitamin supplements can cause depression, anxiety and a whole range of diseases. When taken in excessive amounts vitamins – which many people think of as being entirely harmless – can even kill. In recent years some medical observers have reported that diseases caused by taking too many vitamins are now more common than disorders caused by vitamin deficiency.

Vitamin A taken in excess can produce anorexia, drowsiness, irritability, hair loss, headaches and skin problems. It can also make bones tender and can produce liver damage. The vitamin B group can cause a wide range of problems when taken in excess (despite the fact that, like vitamin C, it is water-soluble and therefore excesses are eventually discarded in the body's wastes). Too much vitamin B3 can cause stomach ulceration, hair loss and liver damage, while too much B6 can cause depression and nerve damage that can lead to clumsiness, numbness and a loss of balance. Too much vitamin C can cause kidney problems – specifically kidney stones – and can affect growing bones. In addition people who have been taking high doses of vitamin C for long periods and then suddenly cut down their intake can develop rebound scurvy. Vitamin D in high doses can cause irreversible damage to the eyes and kidneys by encouraging deposits of calcium, and it can also cause fits, comas, muscular weakness, headaches and high blood pressure. Too much vitamin E can produce a tendency to bleeding when taken with warfarin (a drug commonly prescribed in the treatment of various circulatory disorders). It can also affect immunity levels, reduce sexual function, and produce headaches, eye problems and stomach disorders. An excess of vitamin K can produce a type of anaemia.

The real tragedy is that many of the problems caused by taking too many vitamins (and you don't need to take unduly large doses of supplements to cause problems) are treated as vitamin deficiencies by the individuals concerned. The result, of course, can be a gradual worsening of symptoms.

Minerals can cause trouble too. Zinc, for example, is not as safe as some people claim. The World Health Organization has warned that too high a zinc content can make drinking water dangerous; food poisoning has been produced by storing food in galvanized containers, and children who have chewed metal toys containing zinc have developed a type of anaemia which does not respond to iron treatment. There is even some evidence linking high doses of zinc to the development of high blood pressure.

Everything you need to know about vitamins

Vitamin A

What does it do? Although vitamin A is best known as the vitamin that helps us to see in the dark, this reputation is exaggerated. The rumour is alleged to have originated during the Second World War when it was said that pilots were being fed on carrots (which are rich in vitamin A) so that they would be able to see better during night flying sorties. The truth is not quite so dramatic as this – although vitamin A does help us to see better in dim light, and, because the vitamin is a vital constituent of the pigment visual purple, which is present in the retina, a deficiency can cause night blindness. A shortage of vitamin A is known to cause blindness because of its effects on the cornea and conjunctiva.

Perhaps the most important thing that vitamin A does is to help us fight infection – by keeping our cell walls strong it helps to keep bacteria and viruses at bay. Some researchers do, however, believe that vitamin A deficiency may, in some individuals, lead to the development of certain types of cancer.

What foods contain it? We can obtain vitamin A from some animal foods – liver, eggs and butter are particularly rich in it. Some animal products are, however, so rich in vitamin A that they can be toxic: polar bear liver (not, admittedly a popular delicacy) contains a dangerously high amount. Fish liver oils and margarine also contain useful amounts, as do milk and cheese.

Most of us, however, can obtain all the vitamin A our bodies require from plant foods. Carrots and dark green vegetables are both excellent sources of vitamin A.

Vitamin B1 (thiamine or aneurin)

What does it do? Vitamin B1 helps us to turn the carbohydrates in our food into energy. The amount we need is, therefore, closely related to our intake of carbohydrates – and our need for energy! Absence of B1 produces a typical combination of pins and needles and numbness in the hands and feet; severe deficiency leads to a condition known as beri-beri, which affects the heart and the central nervous system. Beri-beri is common in rice-eating countries where the husk (containing B1) is removed and the rice 'polished'. Our bodies cannot store supplies of vitamin B for long periods, and so a fairly regular intake of this vitamin is essential.

In more developed countries B1 deficiency is common among both alcoholics and elderly people – particularly those who live alone and fail to feed themselves properly. In alcoholics B1 deficiency can lead to permanent brain damage, while in the elderly it more commonly leads to heart disease and mental confusion.

What foods contain it? Vitamin B1 is present in a wide variety of plant foods, but the majority of us get most of our requirement from cereals. As with rice, most of the vitamin is removed from the husk during the milling process, so theoretically white flour should be deficient in vitamin B1. Fortunately, in most countries laws ensure that white flour contains added vitamin B1. Other foods which contain B1 include nuts, beans, eggs and legumes (peas and beans). Some types of meat – particularly pork, ham, bacon, liver and kidneys – contain B1.

Vitamin B2 (riboflavin)

What does it do? Like thiamine (and nicotinic acid or vitamin B3), riboflavin helps us to turn carbohydrate foodstuffs into energy. A deficiency of vitamin B2 is uncommon, but can occur along with a general deficiency of other members of the B group. The usual signs include a sore, discoloured tongue and sore, cracked lips.

What foods contain it? Vitamin B2 is found in some green vegetables and in certain types of meat – particularly liver. Eggs, and dairy products such as milk and cheese, are a rich source. However, it is important to remember that since B2 is sensitive to light, if milk is left in full sunshine on the doorstep its B2 content will be destroyed.

Vitamin B3 (nicotinic acid or niacin)

What does it do? Vitamin B3 has a number of functions. People whose diet contains too little are likely to develop a disease called pellagra which affects the brain, the gastro-intestinal tract and the skin.

What foods contain it? Vitamin B3 is available in a wide variety of plant and animal foods – though never in large amounts. The richest sources of vitamin B3 are wholemeal cereals (the vitamin is removed from white flour during the refining process, but is added again before the white flour is sold); fish and some types of meat (particularly liver) also contain small amounts.

Vitamin B6 (pyridoxine)

What does it do? Although vitamin B6 plays a vital role in the way enzymes metabolize amino acids and proteins, and although some drugs such as oral contraceptives increase the body's requirements for the vitamin, diseases due to vitamin B6 deficiency are not known in adult human beings.

What foods contain it? Although no foods contain large amounts of vitamin B6, many foods contain small amounts – and the body's requirements are only modest. Cereals, fruit and vegetables – and some meats, particularly liver – contain B6. Fairly massive doses of B6 are sometimes prescribed to alleviate premenstrual symptoms, but although there is much anecdotal evidence to support this practice there is little hard evidence. It is important to remember that large amounts of vitamin B6 can cause nerve damage and depression.

Vitamin B12 (cyanocobalamin)

What does it do? Vitamin B12 is, like another micro-nutrient called folic acid, vital for the formation of red blood cells; a shortage of B12 can lead to pernicious anaemia, in which the size of individual red blood cells will be increased but their number reduced. Vitamin B12 plays a part in the functioning of the central nervous system, and a long-term shortage can lead to permanent damage being done to the brain and spinal cord.

B12 is unique in that, before it can be absorbed into the body, it needs to be linked to a substance called an 'intrinsic factor' which is formed in the stomach. Sometimes patients who have had operations on their stomach may be unable to produce this essential 'intrinsic factor'.

Many people who give up eating meat worry about developing B12 deficiency since, as is widely known, the richest sources of this vitamin are animal products. Some authorities still claim that vegetarians should take vitamins B12 supplements, but this is not necessary (see below).

What foods contain it? Liver is by far the commonest source of vitamin B12, but milk, other dairy products and eggs also contain a plentiful supply. Vegans can obtain their B12 from edible seaweeds, tempeh, soya milk and the wide variety of fortified products available, including yeast extracts, cereals, margarines and textured vegetable protein. However, as the B12 used to fortify these vegan foods is quite likely to be of animal origin, some vegans do have to break their own rules in order to stay alive.

Since folic acid is contained in plentiful supplies in green vegetables, even vegans are unlikely to become folic acid-deficient unless they eat a poorly balanced diet.

Vitamin C (ascorbic acid)

What does it do? Vitamin C has a wide variety of tasks. We need a regular supply since, like all the vitamin B constituents, it is water-soluble and therefore not stored in the body. One vital function of vitamin C is to help form connective tissue – the packing material that supports and protects the rest of the body. The skin contains a considerable amount of connective tissue, and a shortage of this vitamin leads to bruising and bleeding. This condition, known as scurvy, is typified by bleeding gums and by the fact that cuts and grazes take an unusually long time to heal. Scurvy still occurs quite commonly – particularly among the elderly and among people who are heavy meat-eaters but who do not eat many vegetables or much fruit.

Vitamin C also helps us to fight infections (though, as I explained earlier, extra doses do not make us any healthier).

Additionally, it helps us to absorb iron – indeed, it increases the ease with which iron is absorbed by a factor of five, and for this reason alone meat-eaters are, ironically, sometimes more likely to develop iron deficiency anaemia than are vegetarians. Finally, it is worth pointing out that women need slightly more vitamin C than men, that smokers need considerably more than non-smokers, and that the sick and convalescent need good quantities of vitamin C too.

What foods contain it? In 1535 Jacques Cartier sailed from St Malo in France with a crew of 110, intending to explore the coast of Newfoundland, but within six weeks one hundred of his men had developed scurvy – caused by the absence of vitamin C from their diet. Luckily for his men and his expedition Cartier discovered from a native that the complaint could be cured by drinking juice from the fruit of local trees. His crew recovered within days. Wise sea captains quickly followed Cartier's example and, to ensure good health on long voyages, made sure that each man was provided with a regular supply of either orange or lemon juice. In a book called *The Surgeon's Mate*, published in 1636, John Woodall recommended these juices for the prevention of scurvy.

Remarkably and inexplicably, sea captains then stopped providing their men with citrus fruits and scurvy began once again to decimate crews on long voyages. When Admiral Anson's fleet went round the world between 1740 and 1744 three-quarters of the men died from the disease. It was not until 1747 that the idea of preventing scurvy by giving sailors lemon or orange juice was reintroduced. The man who suggested it was Dr James Lind, who in this connection performed what was probably the first proper clinical trial. It was his work which enabled Cook to sail around the world between 1769 and 1771 without a single case of scurvy. Surprisingly, however, it was not until 1795 that lemon juice became a compulsory part of every sailor's diet. To make sure that sailors took it, it was added to their grog ration. When in later years limes were used instead of lemons, the Americans gave British sailors the nickname 'limey' to commemorate the fact.

Today it is widely recognized that fresh fruit of most kinds (especially citrus) and fresh vegetables contain good quantities of vitamin C. Amazingly, however, one of the most important sources is the potato – simply because in much of the Western world potatoes make up a large part of the average diet. New potatoes contain more vitamin C than old ones, and overcooking vegetables destroys this vitamin. It is also worth remembering that, since vitamin C is soluble in water, leaving vegetables soaking for a long time will cause the vitamin C to disappear. Chips, by the way, keep their vitamin C – fat 'seals' the vitamin in.

Vitamin D (cholecalciferol)

What does it do? Vitamin D is needed if we are to absorb and use calcium and phosphorus properly for the production of strong bones and teeth. A deficiency causes a condition called rickets in children. It's characteristics are bow legs, swollen knees and swollen wrists; all are caused by a disorder in the way that new bone is formed at the ends of growing bones. In adults a deficiency gives rise to osteomalacia, in which bones become weak and prone to fracture.

What foods contain it? Like vitamins A and E, vitamin D is found in fairly large quantities in animals because they can all be stored. Relatively few foods contain large quantities of vitamin D, but the substances which do contain it include many different types of fish (especially herrings, mackerel and canned sardines and pilchards), eggs and dairy products such as butter, cheese and cream. Cod liver oil also contains it, and there is often added vitamin D in margarine.

To a certain extent all this is irrelevant, since most of us can make all the vitamin D we need from the action of sunshine on our skin. Even in fairly dull, overcast countries the majority of individuals see enough sunshine to produce all the vitamin D that they need.

Vitamin E (tocopherols)

What does it do? Despite the hype that surrounds vitamin E deficiency, disorders are virtually unknown – the only properly recorded deficiency is a type of anaemia in premature babies. Some individuals claim that vitamin E supplements can be used to boost sexual, mental or athletic skills; there is not, however, any scientific evidence to support these outlandish claims. Vitamin E has a rather bloated reputaion as the sex vitamin, but this is based on some experiments done on rats many decades ago – even then the experiments simply showed that a deficiency in rats can lead to sterility. Since a deficiency in humans is virtually unknown (human beings would be dead before they developed vitamin E deficiency) and experiments on animals are of no relevance to human beings, it is doubtful if this early research is now of any significance at all.

What foods contain it? A vegetarian diet is particularly rich in vitamin E since the vitamin is found in vegetable oils and green leafy vegetables. Eggs also contain some vitamin E. If you are eating a reasonably balanced diet, then you are almost certainly getting all the vitamin E your body needs.

Vitamin K (napthoquinones)

What does it do? Vitamin K plays a vital role in the blood clotting mechanism. A shortage can sometimes occur in babies and small children, but it is very rare in adults.

What foods contain it? We can, it seems, make our own vitamin K. Fresh, green, leafy vegetables such as broccoli, cabbage, lettuce and spinach all contain vitamin K. The only type of meat that contains appreciable amounts of this vitamin is liver.

Everything you need to know about minerals

I have already talked about how unnecessary mineral supplements are, and how the public can be deceived by misleading claims from manufacturers into parting with their hard-earned money. The truth about minerals is much simpler, much less dramatic and much less alarming.

Your body *does* need minerals, of course: they perform a wide variety of vital functions. Iron, for example, is essential for the formation of red blood cells; without it your body would form too few red blood cells and your tissues would not receive enough oxygen (the red blood cells carry oxygen around your body – oxygen is needed to produce energy).

Vitamins and minerals

To make sure you get the quantities you need:
- eat a varied diet which includes fresh fruit, green vegetables, peas and beans, wholemeal products and dairy produce
- eat nuts and seeds, which contain a variety of vitamins and minerals and therefore make good nutritional snacks
- throw away aluminium saucepans (aluminium is a potential poison which can cause brain damage) and use iron ones, which can add useful quantities of iron to cooked food
- eat fruit and vegetables in their skins whenever possible – don't peel thickly, since many vitamins are stored just underneath the skin
- steam, stir-fry or microwave vegetables instead of boiling – this helps to preserve water-soluble vitamins (the B group and vitamin C)
- use as little water as possible when boiling vegetables
- cook vegetables for as little time as possible
- prepare food quickly and try not to keep it hot or to reheat it – this can destroy vitamins
- keep milk away from the light – daylight destroys some B vitamins
- remember that skimmed or semi-skimmed milk and low-fat cheeses do contain as much calcium and B vitamin as full cream milk and cheese but less vitamin A and vitamin D (because these vitamins are fat-soluble)
- appreciate that bizarre slimming diets can be dangerously short of essential vitamins and minerals – the *Eat Green* diet will ensure that you receive the vitamins and minerals you need
- eat raw foods whenever you can – vitamins are less likely to be destroyed
- if you suspect that you could be suffering from a vitamin or mineral deficiency see your doctor for advice; never take vitamin or mineral supplements without medical advice

Calcium helps form the structure of bones, and teeth. Zinc is essential for the proper functioning of some of the body's enzymes.

But your body can get all the minerals it needs from a good, regular, balanced diet. If you need minerals for any reason then you *must* see your doctor so that he can ensure you receive the correct quantities of the correct supplements.

And despite the claims made by some 'experts', there is no need for vegetarians to take mineral supplements. There is, for example, iron in dark green vegetables such as cabbage, kale and spinach; in beans and peas; and in dried fruit. The plentiful vitamin C in a vegetarian diet means that the available iron is readily absorbed. Calcium is also available in dark green vegetables, in beans, and in dairy products such as milk and cheese. I'm a vegetarian and I'm well aware of the body's need for minerals, but I never take mineral supplements.

Water

You may not think of water as 'food', but there is no doubt that water is just as valuable as anything we eat. If you had no food to eat and no water to drink, the shortage of water would kill you far more rapidly than the lack of food.

Your water requirements vary according to the outside temperature (when the weather is hot your body deliberately loses water as sweat in an attempt to keep your internal temperature low), but even when the outside temperature is cool some water will be lost in urine, in faeces and by evaporation from your skin. On the other hand your intake of water as fluid will be supplemented by the water present in the foods you eat (some vegetables and fruits are 90 per cent water) and by the fact that the metabolism of carbohydrates, proteins and fat leads to the production of some water. On balance the average-sized individual living in a temperate climate will need at least a litre of fluid a day in order to maintain healthy kidneys and satisfy the body's requirements.

The problem today is finding water fit to drink. Most of us take it for granted that our drinking water is fresh and pure. We turn on the tap and make ourselves a cup of coffee content in the knowledge that the water we're getting has been carefully purified and that all contaminants have been removed. The horrifying truth is that the water most of us get when we turn on our taps contains so many chemicals that it is probably unfit to drink. There are several reasons for this.

Contamination

First, there is the undeniable fact that many of our facilities for extracting and supplying water are archaic. Many water pipes were laid back in the nineteenth century and today there are still thousands of people who get their water supplies pumped through lead pipes. As anyone who works in the water industry will readily confirm, water that passes through lead piping has a nasty tendency to pick up quite a bit of lead before it splutters out of your tap. Lead in drinking water causes many serious problems – including damage to the brain and nervous system.

Second, much of our drinking water is contaminated with nitrates. This problem is created by farmers who use large quantities of artificial fertilizer. The nitrates from the fertilizer seep down into the ground and eventually find their way into the water supplies. Exactly what damage nitrates do to the human body is still something of a mystery, but there is growing evidence linking nitrates to the development of stomach cancer and to circulatory problems in small babies.

'Purification'

The next major problem is that, in their attempts to make our drinking water safe, the people who have the job of looking after it often use chemicals to disinfect, sterilize, purify or cleanse the product they provide. Two of the substances most widely used are chlorine and aluminium sulphate. Those who use these chemicals invariably claim that the substances are safe and that their systems are foolproof. Sadly, the claims are unconvincing.

Already many water authorities around the world have started to cut down on the amount of chlorine they use because of the possible dangers. Scientists now suspect that one of the substances that may be produced when chlorine comes into contact with natural acids in peaty soils could partly explain the recent rise in the incidence of intestinal cancers.

Aluminium sulphate is becoming a major worry too. Aluminium is used partly to help remove the acids that might otherwise interact with the chlorine to create cancer-producing chemicals, and partly to take the discoloration out of peaty water. But people in many areas drink water with aluminium levels that exceed accepted safety limits. The real worry is that there is now evidence linking the drinking of aluminium-rich water to the development of premature senility – and, in particular, Alzheimer's disease. This fear isn't particularly new – the link was first established ten years ago, and since Alzheimer's disease causes a brain disorder indistinguishable from the sort of mental decay associated with great old age, it is difficult to understand how or why the danger was ignored for so long.

As to the claims that the quantities of chemicals used are modest and that the application systems are foolproof – well, those claims have to be put into perspective. We all know that in numerous separate incidents dangerously large quantities of chemicals have been accidentally dumped into drinking water supplies.

Additives

My next worry is that in addition to the chemicals that get into the water by mistake, and the chemicals that are put into the water in an attempt to make it safer to drink, the water authorities are now empowered to put at least one additional chemical into the water to keep us 'healthy'. The substance commonly added to drinking water supplies is fluoride – in the hope that it will help reduce the incidence of tooth decay among children. The link between fluoride and tooth decay was first established at the end of the nineteenth century. In the decades which followed scientists managed to show that fluoride helps to protect teeth by making tooth enamel – the hard outside covering – tougher and more decay-resistant than usual. Tests done on large numbers of people showed fairly conclusively that tooth decay was slower in those parts of the country where drinking water supplies naturally contained fluoride.

It wasn't long before scientists and politicians started to put forward the suggestion that, by putting fluoride into the water supplies in parts of the world where the natural supplies of fluoride are low, it might be possible to improve the dental health of the rest of the community. The fluoridation of water supplies began in America in 1945, and today the move towards fluoridation is spreading all over the world.

Most of the support for this step has come from politicians (who like the idea of cutting health care costs with such a simple, cheap technique) rather than doctors or dentists. And although it is perfectly true that fluoride does help to protect teeth, those who oppose the compulsory fluoridation of water supplies have been able to muster a number of strong arguments in their favour.

First, you don't have to add fluoride to drinking water in order to protect teeth. You can get the same effect by persuading people to use fluoride mouth washes, fluoride tablets or, most practical of all, fluoride toothpastes. Since most of the toothpastes now on sale contain fluoride, there is no doubt that the vast majority of the population get all the fluoride they need simply by brushing their teeth.

Second, putting fluoride into the drinking water supplies is a potentially dangerous business. The amount put into the water has to be judged very accurately: to get the best effect you need about one part per million. Just twice that much can cause mottling of the teeth, forty times as much can cause a rather nasty bone condition, and if the levels rise any higher then there could well be an associated cancer risk (no one really knows what happens when the levels get higher).

The people who are responsible for putting the fluoride into our drinking water claim that the systems they use are foolproof, but there is now plenty of evidence to show that there is no such thing as a 'foolproof' system. Many people have already been poisoned by accidental overdoses of chemicals. It is also worth pointing out that in 1986 the World Health Organization published a report in which concern was expressed about the incidence of dental problems caused by there being too much fluoride in public drinking water supplies. Getting excess fluoride out of the drinking water is extremely difficult.

Third, our water supplies already contain a number of chemicals – nitrates, chlorine and aluminium sulphate are just three of the ingredients in the cocktail that comes out of your tap. Adding fluoride to the mixture means that the danger of new compounds being created increases dramatically. Whenever chemicals exist in solution together, there are chemical reactions. No one really knows what all these added ingredients are likely to do to one another.

The fourth argument against mass fluoridation is based on the fact that a growing number of people now seem to be allergic to the chemicals that are put into our drinking water. Many people are, in particular, allergic to fluoride. Several scientific papers analysing these allergic effects have already been published; in some areas the problems have become so bad that it has been suggested that patients allergic to their own tap water will have to get distilled water on prescription from their doctor.

The final anti-fluoridation argument is based on the fact that, having apparently 'won' the pro-fluoridation battle, some scientists and politicians are already suggesting putting other chemicals into drinking water supplies. So, for example, it has already been suggested that drinking water has antibiotics added to it (to reduce the risk of infection – and thereby cut health costs even more), tranquillizers (to calm us all down and allow the politicians to get on with running the country without so many protests) and contraceptives (to reduce the birth rate).

The drug pollution cycle

My own personal worry about the quality of our water supplies is just as serious. It is, I think, fairly well accepted that the number of people taking prescribed drugs has risen steadily in recent years. Millions of people now regularly take drugs as powerful and as varied as sleeping tablets, steroids for asthma and arthritis, painkillers and contraceptive pills.

Once a drug gets into a human body it will be broken down (metabolized) before being excreted. Many drugs are excreted in the urine. Remarkably, some of the most popularly prescribed drugs leave the body in much the same form as they entered it. For example, 75 per cent of a dose of diazepam (one of the most popularly prescribed tranquillizers) leaves in urine as another version of the drug. A third of a dose of ampicillin (a widely prescribed antibiotic) is excreted in the urine within six hours of the pill or capsule being swallowed. What's true of these drugs is true for many thousands of others.

Once it leaves our homes domestic waste – water and solid sewage – goes to sewage treatment plants where it is 'purified'. Standard technical procedures – many of them devised in the nineteenth century – are used to remove bacteria and other obvious contaminants before the apparently 'pure' effluent is allowed to go back into circulation.

The big problem is, however, that although the obvious waste materials are removed from our water supplies the scientists still haven't worked out a way to get drug and hormone residues out of sewage. So when the allegedly pure domestic waste is put back into our rivers it still contains drug residues – tranquillizers, antibiotics, blood pressure pills, anti-depression pills, sleeping pills, heart pills, contraceptive pills, painkillers and so on. It also contains residues of other chemicals – such as cosmetics, toiletries and some of the products used in the kitchen or garden.

It's what happens next that really worries me. Our water authorities then take water out of the rivers, purify it once more, and recycle it as ordinary drinking water. All this means that when you turn on your kitchen tap and fill your kettle you are getting water that contains secondhand Valium, secondhand heart drugs, secondhand contraceptive pills and so on. And when you, in your turn, go to the loo your urine contains these same drugs, which then circulate through the system again. Each time another human being somewhere in the cycle takes another tablet, the whole problem is made worse.

Our drinking water has, I believe, become so contaminated with secondhand drugs that everyone who drinks water extracted from a river into which sewage effluent has been discharged is effectively taking small quantities of a wide range of prescription drugs. I've read all sorts of scientific papers and talked to numerous people about this problem. But no one really knows how bad it has already become. Remarkably little research has been done to find out just how long these chemical residues last. The small amount that has been done merely confirms my suspicions that we have a real problem to worry about.

Water

What you can do to reduce your risk of being poisoned:

- if you have a small baby, breast feed it for as long as possible
- if you suffer from any bizarre or inexplicable symptoms it could well be the water you are drinking that is making you ill – this is particularly likely to be the case if you have acquired any new and unusual health problems after recently moving house
- if you suspect that your tap water could be a problem, try drinking bottled water to see if your symptoms disappear
- rainwater collected in water butts may be contaminated by micro-organisms and may contain acids acquired from atmospheric pollutants; but the contaminants can usually be destroyed by boiling and the acid pollutants are in my view probably less dangerous than the ones present in tap water (at least you can be fairly certain that no one will have added a ton of aluminium sulphate to your water butt by mistake)
- get your drinking water tested for contaminants – but remember that even modern tests do not always show up all chemical pollutants
- make your voice heard – protest to your political representatives about the poor quality of drinking water supplies; things will only be changed if protests are made

---

For example, when scientists tested river water they found detectable amounts of progestogen (one of the ingredients of the contraceptive pill) in it. Research carried out in Germany has shown that the amount of oestrogen (another ingredient of the contraceptive pill) seems to be increasing in surface water supplies. This problem is international. Could it be that our male population is being slowly but steadily feminized by drinking water that contains female hormones? Is our male population steadily being turned female? What effects do all these hormone residues have on pregnant women – and their developing babies? Are we all being tranquillized and sedated by unavoidable quantities of secondhand tranquillizers and sleeping tablets?

This may sound like science fiction. It isn't. Many other doctors are already worried about these dangers, and are initiating studies designed to show us precisely what is happening. The big snag is that they are unlikely to produce any results for at least another generation. By then it will be too late.

2

Good for Your Health

The dangers of meat

We tend to think of meat as being an essential part of a healthy diet – at least for those who can afford it. As we in the West have become steadily more prosperous, and as our expectations have grown, so our consumption of meat has increased. During the last century our intake of meat – and meat products – has gone up twenty-fold. Families who, a century ago, would have regarded meat as a 'once-a-week' luxury now see it as a daily essential.

In order to cater for this growing demand farmers have had to change the way they work, and as a result the very nature of the meat we eat has also changed dramatically. For example, whereas the fat content of a free-living wild warthog is a modest 1 – 2 per cent, that of a pig bred especially for the meat market will be between 40 and 50 per cent.

The vast majority of independent food experts (the ones who haven't been bought up by big companies or trade organizations) now firmly believe that most of us eat far too much meat. In this chapter I intend to show why we should eat less. It used to be thought that meat was excellent for slimmers because it is high in protein and low in carbohydrate. This assumption has since been proved wrong. Meat — particularly modern meat – is rich in fats, which can ruin any attempt to lose weight. But there's more to it than that.

The health hazards

It is now known that people who eat a diet which contains high quantities of meat are especially prone to suffer from a wide range of disorders. Two of the most important are heart disease and cancer.

The first evidence linking meat to heart trouble appeared shortly after the Second World War. When Norway was occupied by the Nazis, meat and animal products were scarce – especially for the locals; as a result most Norwegians lived on a diet which consisted largely of cereals, fish and vegetables. The number of deaths from heart disease fell by 21 per cent during this time. When, after the war had finished, people started to eat meat again deaths from heart disease returned to their pre-war level.

Since then many other researchers have established a relationship between high meat consumption and a high incidence of heart disease. In New Zealand, where the consumption of meat and dairy products is amongst the highest in the world, the incidence of coronary heart disease is also amongst the highest in the world. In addition there is a considerable amount of obesity in New Zealand.

There are several theories about the links between meat consumption and cancer. One suggestion is that these days meat contains a number of carcinogens. One of the most disturbing pieces of research, conducted some years ago, established that if an animal killed in a slaughterhouse has a developing cancer it is quite possible for whoever eats meat from the dead animal to acquire that cancer. In one experiment it was shown that if chimpanzees were fed from birth with milk taken from cows which had leukaemia, many of the chimpanzees died in their first year of life – of leukaemia. I do not support animal experiments of any kind, but since these experiments have been performed (and the animals have already died) it would be foolish to ignore the results. Since the principle of cross-species infection with cancer has now been established, all meat-eaters should regard their eating habits as extremely dangerous.

It's impossible to prepare a full list of disorders known to be associated with meat but a preliminary list would have to include the following disorders:

anaemia	breast cancer
angina and heart disease	cancer of the colon
appendicitis	cancer of the prostate

constipation
diabetes
gallstones
gout
haemorrhoids (piles)

high blood pressure
indigestion
obesity
strokes
varicose veins

Many of these disorders will improve – or in some cases disappear entirely – if a meat-free or low-meat diet is adopted. This list is not, of course, comprehensive. There are many other conditions which are associated with the consumption of meat. Some disorders – for example tapeworms – are only *ever* found among meat-eaters.

Danger on the farm

Most meat-eaters innocently imagine that when they buy raw meat it is free of all chemicals and artificial additives. Sadly, this is not true. In order to maintain their profits modern farmers use many drugs and artificial chemicals to keep their animals healthy and to improve the weight or appearance of the animals they take to market. The variety of chemicals used varies from farm to farm. Some farmers use tranquillizers to make sure that live animals are little trouble in crowded pens, but the two groups of drugs most widely used are antibiotics and hormones.

Antibiotics are used to reduce the risk of infection which, since animals are expensive to breed, rear and keep, can be a costly disruption to a farming business. In most modern farms animals are kept in absolutely appalling conditions (see page 85). There is little room for movement, and cross-infection is extremely likely. A few years ago antibiotics were used simply to treat sick animals and to prevent illness spreading. Today they are routinely added to animal feeds in order to help prevent infection developing and to encourage a faster average growth rate. Nearly half of all the antibiotics manufactured go into animal feeds. Young animals are taken from their mothers at such an early age that they have no chance to acquire any natural protection by drinking their mother's milk – they are therefore far more susceptible to disease and often need to take antibiotics for life.

The real danger with giving animals antibiotics is that

eventually drug-resistant bacteria will develop; then the antibiotics given to animals will no longer be of any value in the treatment of human infections. To a large extent this is already happening. When humans eat the meat from animals fed on antibiotics, they ingest both the remnants of the antibiotics and the bacteria which have acquired antibiotic resistance. Giving antibiotics to animals may help to improve farmer's profits, but the habit will lead to enormous problems in the future for all those who eat meat.

The use of hormones also presents a serious hazard to human health. Indeed, the danger is so great that in Europe the sale of hormone-treated beef has been officially banned. Sadly, however, the ban is of more academic than practical interest, for the evidence shows that many farmers are still ignoring the ban. In Belgium, for example, it was recently found that as many as one in every four hamburgers contained growth hormones that had originally been given to cattle.

The main reason why farmers like giving hormones to their cattle is a simple one. If you give an animal a growth hormone it will grow faster and achieve a heavier weight sooner.

QUESTION: *Is a vegetarian diet safe for pregnant women?*

ANSWER: *Yes. A properly balanced vegetarian diet is, in fact, less likely to produce nutritional problems than a diet which includes meat.*

One of the hormones commonly used is diethylstilboestrol – popular among farmers because it helps both sheep and cattle to fatten quickly. The problem is that diethylstilboestrol is a dangerous substance. Not long after the Second World War it was prescribed for pregnant women who seemed likely to have miscarriages. Only in the early 1970's, however, was it revealed that daughters of the women who had been given the hormone were prone to develop vaginal cancer. This was the first time in medical history that a drug given to one generation had been shown to cause problems in the next, years after a safe and apparently incident-free birth. Officially, farmers are banned from using diethylstilboestrol, but there is strong evidence to show that they are still using it.

In America the use of hormones to boost the size of animals is commonplace: around four-fifths of all US-raised cattle still get treated with hormones. In a way this dangerous deceit is not surprising. A single, cheap pellet of hormones can make an animal put on an extra 50lb (22kg) of lean meat – while eating less than an animal that hasn't had hormone assistance.

But the human cost could be terrible. The ban on hormones in Europe was decreed in 1980, after Italian mothers had noticed that their babies were developing breasts. They had been given baby food manufactured from animals fed on diethylstilboestrol. More recently doctors in Brazil and Puerto Rico have reported that a number of babies and very young girls have developed breasts, started lactating and begun to menstruate after being fed on milk that has come from animals that have been given hormones.

Despite all this evidence farmers in Europe still spend huge sums of money on illegally purchasing these hormones. There are now fifteen illegal growth hormones available on the black market in Europe, and meat from just about all countries is widely affected.

Antibiotics and hormones are not the only drugs likely to be ingested by people who eat meat. Farmers use a wide range of other products to keep their animals alive – and to ensure that they are acceptably profitable. For example, they sometimes inject substances called prostaglandins into animals to bring them into 'season' at the same time; this is obviously more convenient than waiting for nature to take its course. In addition farmers administer to their animals chemicals which, when ingested, kill any fly eggs which might be laid in manure. This technique is designed to reduce the number of flies in overcrowded animal sheds, but no one yet knows what effect the accumulated toxins might have on human consumers.

In addition to all these chemicals it is also worth remembering that, when eating meat, we also eat whatever other chemicals or 'natural' substances might have accumulated in the animal's body before its death. So, for example, if an animal had a large amount of uric acid in its bloodstream then the people eating its meat will swallow that uric acid. Uric acid can accumulate and lead to the development of gout, arthritis and kidney stones. Finally, when terrified in the slaughter-house animals produce massive amounts of adrenalin. I don't think anyone yet knows just what sort of effect animal adrenalin can have on a human consumer.

Danger in the abattoir

The enormous modern demand for meat means that every day huge numbers of animals are transported to large regional abattoirs to be killed and processed. Theoretically, the process should be clean, hygienic, fast, efficient and painless. It is none of those things.

The very size of the market means that the slaughter goes on in huge sheds where cross-infection is commonplace and where there is little or no time to clear away blood or faecal matter. Chickens are routinely killed in batches of ten thousand at a time, and even fast-flow high-technology meat plants cannot cope with that sort of quantity without carcasses being infected and cross-infected. Everything goes too fast to allow for proper cleaning procedures to be followed, and abattoirs have regularly been criticized by inspection groups for ignoring or overlooking the rules and regulations which are designed to protect both the animals and the consumers.

No one has time to check if any animal has some obscure cancer. No one can rule out the risk of an infected animal infecting thousands of other beasts. Contamination with faecal matter is too commonplace to be remarkable.

Modern regulations allow meat processors and packers to confuse and mislead consumers. The word 'meat' can include the tail, head, feet, rectum and spinal cord of an animal. The term 'meat products' can include the eyeballs and the nose. A package containing 100 per cent pure beef may include heart, fat, skin, rind and gristle. Sausages commonly contain ground up intestines, fat, bone, cartilage and even tonsils. Colourings and preservatives are added to dead carcasses to make meat look more attractive. No one washes off faecal matter – it is left as added weight. Water and polyphosphates are injected into the dead body at high pressure to increase the weight of the meat.

And it isn't just red meat that contains chemicals, pollutants and infective organisms. White meat from chickens and turkeys is just as bad. Most chickens around the world now seem to be infected with salmonella – an infective organism which doesn't normally cause the chicken any great harm and which certainly doesn't affect its profitability. Over half the cases of salmonella affecting humans are believed to have been caused by the consumption of chicken meat.

Danger at home

There is even evidence to show that, if meat is smoked or cooked on a barbecue, those eating it will run an increased risk of developing cancer.

Are you eating your way to illness?

The food you choose to eat can keep you fit, strong and healthy, or it can make you ill. There is no longer any doubt about this; the diet you choose will determine how healthy you are and what disorders you suffer from.

In recent years scientists have accumulated an enormous amount of evidence to show that most of us eat too much fat, meat and sugar and not enough fresh fruit, fresh vegetables and fibre. Tragically, many Western countries have now successfully exported their poor eating habits to under-developed countries. As a result the fortunate few who have survived famine and infection are now succumbing to West-ern-style diseases.

The list of diseases associated with food seems to get longer every year. We now know that the range of disorders associated with the food we eat varies from heart disease and high blood pressure to gall bladder disease and varicose veins. Asthma, allergy problems and many types of cancer are also known to be a result of poor eating habits.

On the following pages I have listed just *some* of the disorders known to be linked to poor eating habits. I don't promise any miracles, but if you follow the eating advice in *Eat Green* you will be far less likely to suffer from these problems, and if you are unfortunate enough to be already suffering from any of them you will almost certainly see a noticeable improvement in your condition if you follow the *Eat Green* eating philosophy.

One word of warning, however. If you are already receiving any medical treatment do please talk to your doctor before changing your eating habits. It is quite likely that if you change your eating habits your need for medical help will change too. So, for example, if you have high blood pressure and you change your eating habits, then your blood pressure may well fall. Your need for medication may vary – or even disappear completely. You will need to see your doctor regularly while you are changing your diet or during any weight loss.

Acne

You can help clear up acne by eating less fat and less sugar and more fibre. Several scientific studies have shown that there are powerful links between eating habits and this common, troublesome and embarrassing skin disorder. For example, it has been shown that Eskimos who change to a Western diet develop more acne than Eskimos who remain faithful to their traditional, natural diet. It has also been shown that there is less acne among black people living in Zambia and Kenya on a traditional diet than there is among black people living in America – the main difference between the two groups is, of course, the diet they eat.

Allergies

Hay fever, eczema, dermatitis and rhinitis – and some varieties of asthma – are frequently caused by allergies. These disorders are now much more common than they were a few decades ago – eczema affected 2 people per 1000 born in 1946 but over 12 per 1000 of the following generation – and are all known to be more common among people who eat a junk food diet or large amounts of dairy food. Sadly, a diagnosis of 'food allergy' has become an easy, vague, 'catch-all' diagnosis. Some unscrupulous health practitioners have been too eager to make this diagnosis whenever difficult symptoms have appeared. But there is no doubt that many people whose diet includes too many refined foods, too many additive-rich foods and not enough fresh fruit or vegetables would be much healthier if they changed their eating habits.

Anaemia

Most people imagine that vegetarians are more prone to become anaemic than meat-eaters. This is no longer true, and today anaemia is probably commoner among meat-eaters than among vegetarians! There are two reasons: first, many meat products contain very few genuinely useful nutritional ingredients; and second, the human body can absorb iron far more readily when a diet is rich in vitamin C. People who eat meat often eat far too little fruit and far too few fresh vegetables.

Anxiety

If you suffer a lot from anxiety, then you may be able to reduce your symptoms by cutting down your caffeine intake and by reducing the amount of sugar you eat. Researchers have also shown that many anxiety sufferers live on a diet which contains too little vitamin B.

Asthma

The incidence of asthma has trebled in the last two or three generations. There seems little doubt that our eating habits are at least partly responsible for this. Research evidence from around the world shows that dairy products – milk, butter and cheese – are particularly likely to cause problems, though a diet that includes too much fatty meat can also cause trouble. Many asthmatics have found that their symptoms improve if they change to a diet based on vegetables, fruit and nuts. Incidentally, in emergencies it is possible to gain some relief by drinking beverages which are rich in caffeine – this powerful drug acts as an effective broncho-dilator. Coffee, tea and cola drinks can all provide short-term relief.

Atherosclerosis

Atherosclerosis – or clogged up arteries – is a frequent cause of heart disease, high blood pressure and strokes. There is ample evidence now available to show that this disorder is closely linked to dietary habits. Eat too much fat (particularly saturated animal fats) or sugar, and your risk of developing atherosclerosis is dramatically increased. There is even some evidence to show that a high caffeine consumption can make problems worse. You can, however, help yourself enormously by eating more vegetables, more high-fibre foods such as oat bran (now known to reduce blood cholesterol levels), more beans, more live yoghurt and more garlic and onions. A modest alcohol intake may also prove helpful.

Cancer

Doctors now estimate that between one-third and one-half of all cancers are associated with the food we eat. Some experts claim that for women the risks are even greater, and that poor eating habits cause or contribute to *more* than half of all cases of cancer. A high fat intake has been linked to an increased incidence of cancers of the breast and the colon; eating cured, pickled and smoked foods is believed to be responsible for many cases of cancer in the stomach and the oesophagus; and a low-fibre, high-fat diet is now believed to be associated with the incidence of ovarian and uterine cancers in women and cancer of the prostate in men.

The safest type of diet if you want to reduce your risk of developing cancer is a 'green' one: more fruit, vegetables and wholegrain cereals, and fewer fatty foods. You should also avoid pickled and smoked foods and drink alcohol only moderately. Researchers now suggest that a 'green' diet helps in several ways; not only are there fewer cancer-inducing chemicals in these foods, but the high fibre component of the diet means that any chemicals which *are* present spend far less time in the body and are less easily absorbed. Finally, there is evidence to show that individuals who are overweight are more likely to suffer from cancer than individuals who are not overweight – and my 'green' diet is, of course, excellent for slimmers.

Cataracts

Reduce your risk of developing a cataract by keeping your intake of sugar low.

Constipation

A diet that contains plenty of fibre (or roughage) will help prevent constipation. The 'green' diet is perfect for anyone who suffers from it.

Depression

Evidence suggests that people who suffer from depression should try to include plenty of fresh fruit in their diet – and to eat a good supply of foods rich in vitamin B. The 'green' diet is perfect.

Diabetes

Cutting down on sugar and fat will help people not to develop diabetes; it will also assist many who have already become diabetics to avoid the need for treatment. The 'green' diet, low in fat and sugar and high in fibre and complex carbohydrates, is excellent. The fibre helps by slowing down the rate at which sugar is absorbed, and the slimming effect of the diet is also useful.

Gall bladder disease (including gallstones)

There is no doubt at all that the high incidence of gallstones in our society is closely linked to our dietary habits. We eat too much fat, we eat too little fibre and our intake of calories is far too high – gallstones are an almost inevitable consequence. The risk of developing or exacerbating gallstones can be dramatically reduced by avoiding refined carbohydrates, avoiding fats of all kinds, avoiding or dealing with being overweight, and increasing one's intake of fibre-rich fruit, vegetables and wholegrain cereals. There is also evidence that eating a regular breakfast helps to reduce the risk of gall bladder trouble developing.

Finally, some experts have shown that food allergies can sometimes lead to gall bladder problems. The three foods most likely to cause trouble are eggs, pork and onions. Those suffering from gall bladder disorders should dramatically reduce their intake of these three foods – or try cutting them out altogether for a while to see if their symptoms disappear entirely.

Gout

To conquer gout – or avoid it – restrict your intake of alcohol and drastically reduce the amount of meat you eat. It may also help to limit your intake of fish, peas and beans.

Headaches

Apart from stress, tension and anxiety, foodstuffs are the commonest cause of headaches. Many regular headache sufferers get problems because of a sensitivity to particular types of food. Chocolate, alcohol, fatty foods and additive-rich foods are among the most frequent culprits. Some patients have been able to deal with their headaches permanently by keeping a diary, finding out which foods seem to trigger their symptoms, and then eliminating them from their diet. Many patients find that their headaches are caused by caffeine: in some cases the symptoms are caused when too much caffeine is drunk; in others, headaches appear as withdrawal symptoms.

Heart disease

I've dealt with this subject at some length on pages 29 – 34 and 69 – 70

High Blood Pressure

Numerous surveys have now shown that many people who suffer from high blood pressure can control their problem without pills — simply by managing their diet more thoughtfully. In general a low-fat, high-fibre 'green' diet will help their alcohol and salt consumption to the minimum and by increasing their intake of potassium. The evidence now available shows that anyone who has high blood pressure (or who has a family history of high blood pressure) should reduce his or her salt intake by avoiding the following (or, at least, keeping their consumption as low as possible):

processed foods in general
canned foods
junk foods (such as take-
away hamburgers)
crisps
salted peanuts

salted biscuits
salted butter
salted cheese
sausages
bacon

Salt should not be added to foods that are being cooked, and the salt cellar should be banished from the table. Other flavourings which can be used instead of salt include lemon juice, parsley, garlic, horseradish and tarragon.

Just as there is evidence that too much salt has an adverse effect on patients with high blood pressure, there is also evidence that some patients with blood pressure problems are deficient in potassium. Foods that are rich in potassium include:

apples	dates
apricots	grapefruit
asparagus	oranges
avocados	peas
bananas	peppers
beans	prunes
brussels sprouts	potatoes
cabbage	radishes
corn on the cob	raisins

Indigestion

To deal effectively with indigestion, try to find out what sort of foods upset your stomach most — and avoid them. Fried and fatty foods are most likely to cause problems — although some people do have trouble with specific vegetables such as brussels sprouts, cucumber and radishes. On the whole a low-fat diet will help.

Infections

You can help your body fight off infections more effectively by eating a low-fat, low-cholestrol, low-sugar diet, while at the same time increasing your intake of foods which are naturally rich in vitamins A, B group and C. The 'green' diet is excellent for this purpose. There is now also growing evidence to show that garlic and live yoghurt will help fight off infection.

Insomnia

To sleep better, avoid caffeine and cow's milk and drink very little alcohol.

Irritable bowel syndrome

Astonishingly, experts now believe that one in seven people

in developed countries suffer from the irritable bowel syndrome. The commonest symptoms are abdominal pain together with alternating diarrhoea and constipation. These symptoms can be eased and sometimes eradicated by avoiding sugar and fats and gradually increasing the amount of fibre eaten. (It is important to increase fibre intake only slowly, since too rapid an increase can lead to short-term problems with wind.)

Kidney stones

Avoiding sugar and meat and following a high-fibre, vegetarian diet will help reduce your risk of developing kidney stones. The 'green' diet is well suited to anyone who suffers from this particular problem. Experts also suggest avoiding milk and caffeine and drinking plenty of water.

Multiple sclerosis

A low-fat diet can help multiple sclerosis sufferers. Patients may also be able to help themselves by avoiding foods to which they believe they may be sensitive.

Premenstrual syndrome

Women who suffer from unpleasant, uncomfortable or painful symptoms just before a period may be able to help themselves by reducing their intake of caffeine, milk, salt and sugar. The 'green' diet should prove especially helpful.

Restless legs

This common problem which mostly affects women and usually occurs at night — can usually be controlled by dramatically reducing the intake of caffeine.

Rheumatoid arthritis

Arthritis can be helped by following a low-fat diet. The 'green' diet is excellent for arthritis sufferers, although some experts claim that the amount of fresh fruit eaten should be carefully limited.

Strokes (cerebrovascular disease)

To cut down your risk of having a stroke, eat more fresh

fruit, fresh vegetables and fibre-rich cereals, and avoid foods that are rich in fat.

Tinnitus

This exceptionally annoying problem can be eased by eating a low-fat, low-sugar 'green' diet.

Tooth decay and gum disease

Today half of all five-year-old children in the West have some tooth decay. The world's huge food conglomerates have successfully overcome good eating campaigns supported by dentists and doctors by spending millions on clever advertising designed to encourage children to eat more sweets and chocolates. The constant consumption of sugar-rich foods 'feeds' the bacteria which produce the acid which then attacks teeth and starts the process of decay. By eating fewer sugar-rich foods and by increasing your consumption of fresh fruit and vegetables you will be able dramatically to reduce the risk of suffering from either tooth decay or gum disease.

Ulcers (gastric and duodenal)

The 'green' diet won't miraculously 'cure' an ulcer (there are too many other factors — including stress) but there is evidence to show that it will help.

Varicose veins

We now have proof that the development of varicose veins is associated with a high-fat, low-fibre diet. The 'green' diet will help prevent the development of varicose veins. Constipation and obesity — both problems associated with a high-fat, low-fibre diet — dramatically increase the risk of varicose veins developing.

Why you should buy organic food

These days meat and meat products aren't the only types of food which contain toxins, poisons and potentially harmful additives. Many canned and prepared vegetables and fruits are contaminated with chemicals. Indeed, sometimes apparently *fresh* fruit and vegetables may be contaminated too. During the last few years an increasing number of farmers and market gardeners have attempted to improve their output — and therefore their profits — by using chemicals of many kinds.

Farmers may claim that the chemicals they use are safe, but that simply isn't true. You only have to look at the warning labels on the containers these chemicals come in to realize how potentially dangerous they are. There is much confusion about just how common chemical poisoning is these days. Doctors don't often consider the possibility of a patient with serious or strange symptoms suffering from any sort of poisoning. And yet in America it has been estimated that *at least* one in every two hundred cases of cancer has been caused by pesticides. Astonishingly, there is now evidence to show that 30 per cent of insecticides, 60 per cent of herbicides and 90 per cent of fungicides could cause tumours in human beings. This is no longer a remote or theoretical risk.

The fifteen foods most likely to contain toxic pesticides are, starting with the worst:

1	tomatoes	9	wheat
2	beef	10	soya beans
3	potatoes	11	beans
4	oranges	12	carrots
5	lettuce	13	chicken
6	apples	14	corn
7	peaches	15	grapes
8	pork		

It is fairly clear from this list that you cannot reduce your exposure to dangerous chemicals simply by avoiding meat and meat products — many essential fruits and vegetables are also contaminated.

Pesticides aren't the only source of trouble. In the last few years the use of nitrate fertilizers has rocketed. However, the nitrates they have used are dangerous in two separate but important ways. First, they have contaminated much of our drinking water (see page 54). Second, many foodstuffs now have a dangerously high nitrate content. There is, almost inevitably, a seemingly incontrovertible link between nitrates and cancer.

The only way to avoid eating products contaminated by pesticides and fertilizers is to eat food that has been grown organically — without the aid of any chemicals. More and more people who are 'eating green' are doing just this.

The only snag is that organically grown food doesn't always look as attractive as food that has been grown with the aid of a full range of chemicals. Fruits aren't always the same perfect, predictable shape and vegetables aren't always entirely free of caterpillar holes. Even the colour of food grown organically isn't always quite so bright. On the other hand food grown organically isn't only safe — it is also much better for you (it usually contains more vitamins and minerals) and tastes much better too.

Much the same is true of free-range eggs — eggs laid by chickens which have continuous access to open air runs and which are not cooped up like battery hens. Hens which are cooped up in tiny cages become unhealthy — so they are often given drugs to keep them alive (and laying) longer. In addition, chicken farmers often give chemicals to their hens to make their eggs a deeper yellow (for some reason many consumers prefer to buy eggs which have artificially bright yolks) or to make the shells brown (there is no real difference between a brown-shelled egg and a white-shelled egg but the brown-shelled ones seem to sell much better). Free-range eggs, on the other hand, are not usually contaminated with drugs or chemical additives.

The truth about food additives

Food manufacturers use colourings, flavourings, preservatives and so on to restore or improve the colour, taste or texture of the foods they sell. Altogether they use about 3500 different additives, and in the last few years there has been a considerable amount of discussion about the safety of these substances. The average consumer eats around 5½lb (2.5kg) of additives every year, and many critics have suggested that they may be the cause of a wide range of health problems.

I believe that far too many additives are used — and that

some may well prove to be dangerous. But I also feel that the controversy about additives has been stoked up by journalists and health care practitioners who haven't always told the entire truth. Here, therefore, are the facts you really ought to know about food additives.

QUESTION: *I like the taste of meat. I find the taste of vegetables and bread rather lacklustre. Will I ever really enjoy a vegetarian diet?*

ANSWER: *Yes. Modern meat products and refined foods are full of additives designed to give them extra taste. Many of the products you buy off the supermarket shelf contain fairly large quantities of both sugar and salt (just look at the labels on a few packets and tins – you'll be surprised!). The result is that our taste buds expect strongly flavoured foods. When you stop eating meat and junk foods you will 'miss' the strong, artificial flavours for a while. But gradually you will get your natural sense of taste back. Gradually you will begin to enjoy the real taste of the food you eat.*

Incidentally, if you find the taste of bread rather lacklustre I suspect it is because you are eating refined, packaged, sliced white bread. Try buying a loaf of wholemeal bread or a French stick – you'll quickly taste the difference. Real, fresh bread has a wonderful taste.

What types of additives are there?

Colourings These are included to make food look more attractive. Without colourings frozen peas would look grey rather than green. Some colourings are used deliberately to deceive consumers – for example, meat packers will use a red dye to disguise fat and other non-meat ingredients in pies and sausages.

On the other hand some dyes are used more out of habit than anything else – custard, which consists mainly of corn starch flavoured with vanilla, is coloured yellow because when it was first introduced the aim was to pretend that the product was made from eggs. I doubt if many people still believe that custard powder is made from eggs, but the yellow colouring is still used because consumers *expect* custard to be yellow. No company dares to make a custard powder without the dye, because they know that if they did they would lose all their sales to their competitors.

Flavourings These are used to give extra or added flavour to foods – and sometimes to give an entirely different flavour to a rather bland product. For example, monosodium glutamate is often used to stimulate the taste buds and increase the sensation of flavour. Flavourings are not regulated and there is no permitted list. Strangely, they don't usually have to be named on food labels. Through the skilful use of flavourings just about anything can be made to taste good, for they enable food manufacturers to bulk out foods with wastes or even water.

Preservatives These are used so that foods will last longer without 'spoiling' or 'going bad'. Some preservatives are included to stop colourings and flavourings going off or fading, but most are there to stop micro-organisms developing and turning a product rancid.

Emulsifiers and stabilizers Emulsifiers are used so that water can be bound into a product (usually meat) in order to increase its weight and to give it a smooth firm texture. Stabilizers, often used together with emulsifiers, are there to stop water and fat separating.

The rest Many food additives are used to make foods easier to handle, process or pack. Some are present to improve the consistency of a food – for example, to make a product easier to spread. Anti-splattering agents are sometimes added to oil so that it doesn't splash out of the pan when wet chips are added. Through the skilful use of additives, manufacturers can make products masquerade as things they aren't: for example, additives can be used to make foods *look* like meat or cheese. There is no doubt at all that additives enable manufacturers to debase foods in order to save money.

What harm can additives do?

Quite a lot – but probably not as much as you might imagine. Over the last few years many critics have complained that food additives are responsible for a wide range of disorders. There is little doubt that they *can* cause trouble. They can kill vitamins, for example, and they are now associated with asthma; eczema, dermatitis and other skin rashes; migraine; hyperactivity in children; dizziness; kidney problems; palpitations; diarrhoea; fits; stomach pains and intestinal disorders; as well as many allergy problems. But the dangers have been exaggerated.

One of the commonest complaints is that food additives are responsible for many allergy problems and that, in particular, they commonly cause hyperactivity in children. The link between additives to hyperactivity was first mooted in the 1970's, but since then no doctor has been able to produce clear-cut evidence substantiating this claim. It seems that if there is a link it is likely to be a relatively slight one — with considerably fewer than 1 in 1000 people being affected. Similarly, stories linking additives to cancer have also been exaggerated. Some additives have, it is true, caused cancer in laboratory animals, but there is still no evidence linking additives to humans.

Despite these exaggerations — and my reassurances — I do feel that we all need to take the hazards associated with food additives far more seriously. Many of the most commonly used artificial additives have *never* been tested to see if they are safe for human consumption. Those working in the food industry excuse this bizarre fact by pointing out that there are several thousand additives in use and that testing procedures are lengthy, time-consuming and expensive! This hardly seems to me an adequate excuse for doing nothing.

Nor do I really find it particularly reassuring when food company executives say that 'only' 1 in 1000 people are likely to suffer health problems caused by food additives. We *all* eat food, and therefore if 1 in 1000 people are affected the total number of people involved must be horrifyingly large.

Finally, I find it particularly worrying that so many different additives should be used together. It is widely acknowledged that chemicals frequently interact. If you include two different chemical substances in one product, there is a real risk that the two will combine and produce a chemical change. And modern foods, of course, contain so many different additives that one meal can easily contain fifty different chemicals! No one knows what all those additives are likely to do to one another – or what long-term side-effects may be building up.

Are foods containing only 'natural' ingredients safer than foods that contain additives?

Not necessarily: it depends on what you mean by 'natural'. Over the last few years the food industry has managed to devalue the word 'natural' to such a point that it has become virtually meaningless. For example, food companies will put the magic phrase 'no artificial additives' or the equally reassuring statement 'only natural ingredients' on their labels when the additives they have used are chemicals that occur in nature (or synthetic versions of chemicals which occur in nature) though not necessarily food substances. On the other hand some essential nutrients such as vitamins and minerals sometimes have to be listed as 'additives' as though they were artificial!

So what's the answer?

I suggest that whenever possible you try to buy as many 'fresh' foods as you can. When you need to buy processed and packaged foods, select products that contain a relatively short list of additives. Remember that the substance named first on the packet is the one that appears in the largest quantity inside the packet – other products appear on the list in decreasing order of quantity. Get into the habit of buying from shops or stores that you trust, grow as much of your own food as you can (or buy or 'swop' foods with friends). If you or any member of your family develops hitherto unexperienced symptoms of ill health after buying a new product, try doing without it for a while to see if the symptoms disappear. Finally, you can take considerable comfort from the fact that once you follow the *Eat Green* diet and philosophy you will probably be eating far fewer unnecessary – and potentially unpleasant – additives than you were when you ate meat and meat products.

Eat green and avoid bugs

Despite the widespread use of preservatives and other chemicals designed to help keep food in good condition, there has in recent years been a noticeable and disturbing increase in the incidence of food-borne infections. Vomiting, diarrhoea and stomach pains – typical symptoms of a food-borne gastrointestinal infection – are now commonplace. Food-transmitted infections are so widespread today that no one keeps a strict check on the number of people involved. So I'm delighted to be able to say that here is yet another advantage of choosing to 'eat green'!

The majority of food-borne infections are transmitted via meat and meat products. People who eat a vegetarian or semi-vegetarian diet are far less likely to contract an infection from something they've eaten than are individuals who eat meat.

Meat and meat products are much more likely to be contaminated with infective organisms when they are put on sale, and are considerably more likely to become infected before being eaten.

The risks associated with vegetarian products are slight. You can reduce the risks still further by following this advice:

1 Never buy anything from a shop that looks dirty – or one staffed by people with dirty hands and fingernails. If a shopkeeper can't be bothered to keep his shop – and himself – clean, then the chances are that he can't be bothered to keep the food he sells clean either.

2 Always check the 'sell-by' dates on packaged foods. Don't buy tins which are bulging or rusty. Don't buy packets that are torn or damaged. If you are buying from a freezer, check that the freezer is working and the food is cold when you buy it.

3 Try to buy free-range eggs. If possible, check that the hens from which you buy the eggs are free of salmonella. Don't buy cracked eggs.

4 When you buy chilled or frozen food, take it home as quickly as you can. Carrying food around in a warm car can encourage the growth of bacteria. If possible, take a 'cool box' with you to the shop or supermarket. Put perishable goods in the fridge or freezer as soon as you get home.

5 Check that your fridge is cold enough. The temperature inside should be below 4°C (41°F). If your fridge is too warm, food will spoil — adjust the thermostat if necessary. Defrost your fridge regularly to keep it cooler and more efficient.

6 Take care how you store food in the fridge. Keep different types of food separate to avoid cross-contamination. Always put meat and any foods which are defrosting on a plate at the bottom of the fridge — so that any drips cannot pass on possible infection to other foods. Keep meat — a high-risk source of infection — away from other foods.

7 Always make sure that frozen meat is completely thawed before you start to cook it. This is particularly important for poultry. If you don't take care, there is a risk that when you start to cook the centre of the chicken (or joint) will still be frozen. As a result, when you think the whole piece of meat is cooked the centre will simply be an incubator for bugs.

8 Never refreeze food which has been frozen and already thawed. Thawing increases the number of bacteria.

9 Once food has been thawed use it quickly — don't leave it lying around, or else bugs will have a superb opportunity to multiply.

10 Keep the worktops and utensils in your kitchen clean — use hot soapy water to wash them. Dry them after washing. Remember that cloths can carry — and pass on — germs. Use disposable paper towels to minimize the risk of cross-infection.

11 When preparing food, wash knives and chopping board at regular intervals. Don't use the same knife and board for cutting raw heat and raw vegetables.

12 Wash vegetables, fruit and salads thoroughly — preferably in running water.

13 Wash your hands thoroughly before you start preparing food and after every interruption. After handling meat, poultry or fish, wash your hands again before touching other foods. If you have any infection on your hands be sure to wear an effective bandage — both to protect yourself and the food you are handling.

14 Remember that household pets — cats, dogs and birds — can all carry infections which are dangerous to humans. Keep them away from food and surfaces used to prepare food. Wash your hands thoroughly if you have been handling an animal

---

and intend to prepare food. Keep their feeding dishes and serving utensils separate from yours, and always wash them up separately.

15 The best way to kill bugs in meat, poultry or fish is to cook it properly. Don't eat dishes made of raw meat, poultry or fish.

16 When food has been cooked, eat it immediately. If cooked foods are allowed to cool, bugs can begin to multiply again. The longer cooked food is left, the greater the risk of infection.

17 If you want to store cooked foods to eat later – or you want to keep leftovers – then you should store them carefully: either in very hot conditions or, more likely, in the fridge. Don't put too much warm food into a refrigerator, or the internal temperature of the fridge will rise to unsafe levels.

18 Thoroughly reheat cooked foods before eating. To reheat properly, all parts of the food must reach at least 70°C (158°F).

19 Don't eat dishes prepared with raw eggs, and if you are pregnant, elderly or frail avoid soft cheeses (such as Brie and Camembert) and blue-veined cheeses since these can be contaminated with listeria bacteria.

20 Always follow the instructions carefully if using a microwave. Check your fridge twice a week, and throw out any food that has been in there for too long or that looks to be of doubtful purity. Remember that the signs of food poisoning (vomiting, diarrhoea and abdominal pain) can occur between one hour and five days after eating contaminated food. If you think you have contracted food poisoning rest, avoid solids, drink plenty of fluids and contact your doctor for advice.

3
Good for Your Soul

In addition to all the advantages associated with the 'green' diet, I have no doubt that if you choose to follow the advice in this book you will be making a significant contribution towards making the world a better place to live in. I also have no doubt that if you 'eat green' you will feel better and happier as well as healthier. Knowing that your dietary habits are leading neither to animal suffering nor to starvation in other, less fortunate parts of the world you will feel more at peace with yourself than ever before.

Save animals by eating green

I never used to think very much about the animals we eat. I didn't really associate a chunk of meat with a cow or a piece of veal with a calf. I didn't associate a plump pork sausage, sizzling on the barbecue with a pig. If I thought about the animals I ate, then I believed that they were probably kept in good, clean conditions and killed quickly and humanely. I was wrong – sadly, terribly wrong.

Every single day hundreds of millions of animals and birds suffer so that human beings can eat meat. Chickens are kept in cages so small that they cannot spread their wings. To prevent overcrowded chickens pecking each other to death, farmers hack off the ends of their beaks. Pigs spend their lives confined in narrow stalls or shackled to the floor in conditions which would make anyone with a heart want to weep. Sheds are cramped and filthy, conditions cold and cruel. There are no opportunities for animals to exercise or even to turn around. Calves are taken from their mothers shortly after they are born and are reared in narrow crates; fed on an unnatural, all-liquid diet so that their flesh remains white and plump. Drugs are used to keep these unfortunate creatures alive long enough to reach a certain weight before being bundled off to the slaughterhouse. And next time you pass a lorry carrying live animals or chickens take a closer look. You will, I promise, be horrified and ashamed.

Animals are sensitive creatures. We have a responsibility to care for them properly, but we ignore that responsibility. Two hundred years ago African men and women were captured, taken to America and sold into slavery. In Australia white settlers hunted down the Aboriginals and killed them like vermin. Today we find all that inexplicable, reprehensible and unforgivable. How, I wonder, will our descendants regard our treatment of the animal world?

Every day millions of animals and birds are killed in slaughterhouses. They are not killed cleanly, quickly and painlessly. They suffer.

Young calves stand in their own blood and in the blood of their brothers and sisters. They stand lonely and frightened. But they will still trust humans so much that they will suck at a passing human hand for comfort and love. They are killed crudely and inefficiently, moved from one point to another with the aid of electrical prods; they stand for hours without food; still conscious, they have their throats slit and stand for a

---

QUESTION: *Isn't it true that, if farmers didn't keep animals for us to eat, some breeds would disappear entirely from the face of the earth?*

ANSWER: *According to that theory, the horse ought to have been made extinct by the invention of the internal combustion engine. The truth is that, if agricultural land was used for the production of crops designed for human (rather than animal) consumption, there would be plenty of land to spare on which animals whose purpose was to produce wool, eggs and milk could be allowed to graze naturally. But even if some breeds did disappear I think that would be preferable to our keeping them alive in terrible circumstances.*

---

few moments while their blood pours out. The noise is horrendous. They die in terror, in sadness and in pain. Their killing is merciless and inhumane.

The whole miserable business of preparing animals for the dinner table begins with conception. Artificial insemination is now commonplace – it is cheaper and more reliable. Particularly good breeding cows are used as embryo farms – with the developing calves being transferred to less naturally receptive animals. Geneticists are constantly looking for new ways to improve the quality and size of existing stock.

The bond between mother and baby is as strong among farm animals as it is among humans, but it is ignored by modern farmers. Weaning takes place as early as possible. As soon as a cow can no longer bear calves she will be sent off to be turned into sausages. Recently a cow deprived of her newborn calf escaped from captivity and walked seven miles to find the animal from which she'd been separated at the local market.

Every day tens of millions of one-day-old male chicks are killed because they will not be able to lay eggs. There are no rules about how this mass slaughter takes place. Some are crushed or suffocated to death. Many are used for fertilizer or are fed to other animals.

All around the world animals of every variety are used for food. Dogs, horses, lambs, pigs, cows, goats – the list is endless. Too often those who rear the animals we eat treat them without affection or respect. Everyone conveniently forgets that animals feel both physical and mental pain. Farmers and consumers ignore the fact that no animal wants to die.

Those who farm animals – and sell meat – often claim that because humans are superior to all other species there is nothing wrong with our breeding, killing and eating animals. We can, they claim, do whatever we like with inferior creatures. This seems to me a strange and hollow argument. Surely our ability to think – to imagine and to discuss moral arguments – means that we have an obligation to animals. Besides, if we accept this simple but cruel argument how long will it be before the 'best' and 'brightest' humans start to use the mentally or physically inadequate for experimental fodder – or, horror of horrors, for food? How would we feel if Martians arrived on earth, decided that we, as humans, were less intelligent than they and therefore suitable to use as food? Often, despite the drugs with which they are fed almost daily throughout their lives, animals die before they can be turned into food. It is all a matter of commerce. The cost of breeding replacement stock is less than the cost of looking after animals carefully or providing them with adequate space. The whole sorry business is deeply depressing. Animals which are a year old are often far more rational and sensible than are six week old babies. So, why don't we eat babies? Pigs are as intelligent as cats and dogs and are closer to humans in physiology and anatomy than almost any other animals. And yet we treat pigs with contempt. A pig in close captivity recently undid a bolt to

---

QUESTION: *What about plants? They are alive too, and many studies have shown that by talking to them it is possible to encourage growth. Prince Charles is said to talk regularly to the plants in his garden. If eating animals is wrong, then surely eating plants is wrong too?*

ANSWER: *This is a problem which every vegetarian faces eventually – either because they think of it themselves or because it is put forward by someone else. There are, indeed, some people (fruitarians – see page 14) who eat nothing but the fruits made by plants – and who avoid eating any living plant tissue. My personal answer is that plants have no nervous systems and no brains. I firmly believe that animals suffer terribly when kept in cramped conditions or when brutally killed. But I don't believe that plants suffer in the same way. A rabbit, a pig or a cow can all feel pain – and all have to suffer pain for us to eat them. But I don't believe that a lettuce suffers pain when it is growing or when it is picked. The simple truth is that we've got to eat something, and I find it far more acceptable to eat beans and potatoes than to eat pigs and cows. As always, every individual has to make up his or her own mind about what is right and what is acceptable.*

---

escape from its pen and then liberated other pigs in the same 'factory' by opening their pens too. Can there be any doubt about the intelligence of these creatures? Scientists daily accumulate new evidence proving that all the animals we eat have a complex social life. The law protects dogs and canaries from cruelty but gives not a fig for animals being reared as food.

The final, simplest truth of all is that we do not need to eat animals to stay alive. Animals are bred and killed for the producers' profit and for our pleasure in eating them. I suspect that you will feel more at peace with yourself knowing that you haven't contributed to the torture and destruction of animals. Those of us who eat meat cannot escape responsibility for what is done in our name.

And save the world

It may sound like an exaggeration, but it isn't! By choosing to follow a 'green' diet you will be making a real contribution to the lives of millions of people who daily face starvation. Keeping animals for food is dreadfully wasteful. The average farm animal consumes 20lb (9kg) of plant protein for each 1lb (0.5kg) of meat that it produces. At a United Nations conference on World Hunger a few years ago, Senator Hubert Humphrey pointed out that if each American ate one less hamburger a week then 10 million tons of grain would be made available for the starving world! *That's* how significant your decision to 'eat green' will be.

Eating meat just doesn't make any sense at all in our over-crowded world. Consider these facts:

- Every six seconds someone in the world starves to death. That means that every year around 3½ million people die because they haven't got enough to eat.
- Feeding cereals to animals so that the affluent can eat meat condemns the poor in developing countries to death by starvation.
- Every year approximately 440 million tons of grain are fed to livestock – so that the rich of the world can eat meat. At the same time 500 million people in poorer countries of the world don't have enough to eat.
- India, Thailand and Brazil – countries where thousands have too little to eat – all grow soya which is exported to feed animals in Europe.

- Forests in Brazil are currently being destroyed so that farmers there can graze more cattle – and produce more beef for the American hamburger industry. The destruction of the rain forests doesn't just mean that animals and plants must die. It also interferes with the amount of oxygen in the air and with the world's climate.

- Eating animals means that huge areas of land are used for growing grain to feed the animal population – instead of growing grain to feed people directly. A country as small as Britain could grow enough food for a population of 250 million if they were all vegetarians.

- If we eat the plant protein we grow – instead of feeding it to animals and then eating the animals – the world's food shortage will disappear virtually overnight.

- Ethiopia – home for millions who are starving to death – exports food to the developed world so that the rich can eat meat.

- Farmers in African countries are being encouraged to start poultry and beef farms – even though this will inevitably exacerbate the food shortage in those countries.

- America – which has a modest 6 per cent of the world's population – uses up a massive and greedy 35 per cent of the world's resources.

- In America the average individual consumes around 300lb (135kg) of meat a year. Livestock in America consume most of the country's production of grain, fish and vegetables.

- The world's fresh water shortage is being made worse by animal farming. Farmers use up to eight times as much water preparing animals for the table as they would preparing vegetables and cereals.

- The waste from the world's millions of farm animals pollutes the environment – and, in particular, pollutes water supplies.

- Because we have to grow an enormous amount of grain to feed our animals we have to use fertilizers and pesticides – which damage our health and ruin the environment.

- It is pointless and futile for the world's rich to send cash towards feeding the world's deprived and under-privileged but to continue to eat meat. Remember that 100 acres (40ha) of land will produce enough beef for twenty people, enough wheat for 240 and enough soya beans for 610!

Now do you see why I say that your decision to 'eat green' may help to save the world?

4

Good for Your Shape

Eat green – get slim

At least nine out of every ten people who go on a diet to lose weight will fail. They do so for two reasons.

First, they fail because their 'normal' daily diet is meat-based. They don't feel that they've had a proper meal unless they've eaten some meat or a meat product. In addition, their 'normal' diet probably includes a large number of heavily refined products and relatively few completely natural 'green' products.

Second, when they want to lose weight they invariably choose a boring, unsatisfying and unnatural slimming diet. It's probably difficult to follow. It's probably complicated. It may well be expensive. After a few weeks they feel unsatisfied and maybe even unhealthy. They give up their diet and revert to their original eating habits. Inevitably, they quickly put back on any weight that they've managed to lose.

Once you decide to start 'eating green' – whatever shade of green you choose – your success is guaranteed. Your weight loss will be natural; it will be healthy; and it will be permanent. It's as easy to lose weight on my 'green' diet as it is difficult to lose weight on a meat-based one.

Later on in this book I'll show you exactly how you can follow a 'green' diet easily and without any strain. I'll tell you which foods to eat and show you some of the exciting recipes that you can use. But before that I want to share with you some of the secrets of dieting success.

I've spent much of my life working with slimmers. For many years I was medical adviser to a large and very successful group of slimming clubs and medical consultant to one of the world's most successful slimming magazines. I received thousands of letters from women — and men — who desperately wanted to lose weight, who had tried many times and who just didn't understand why their dieting attempts had so often ended in dismal failure. I now know the secrets of slimming success. I know how you can lose weight easily, healthily and permanently.

You can, of course, skip the next few chapters if you like — and move straight on to Part Three. You'll lose weight — and you'll lose weight steadily and for ever. But if you want to lose weight even faster then I suggest you *don't* skip the next few chapters, because you'll learn a great deal about yourself and about why your previous attempts at dieting haven't worked.

The simple truth is that most of the problems slimmers face are caused by bad habits. People who are overweight tend to eat the wrong foods at the wrong times and for the wrong reasons. By deciding to 'eat green' you will, of course, solve the first problem. With just a little extra effort you can solve the other two major problems as well! You will never find it easier to get rid of all your bad eating habits than you will during the next few weeks while you learn to 'eat green'. Take advantage of the fact that you are changing the way you eat to get rid of *all* the poor eating habits that have given you a weight problem, and you'll lose your unwanted weight even faster.

PART TWO
LOSING WEIGHT —
THE SECRETS OF
SUCCESSFUL SLIMMING

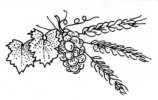

5

Facing the Problem

Overweight – the dangers

Overweight is the biggest problem of the twentieth century – at least one in three of us needs to lose weight. Being fat (there doesn't seem to be any point in avoiding the word – euphemisms merely disguise the nature of the problem, they don't eradicate it) makes people miserable; it makes diseases as varied as asthma and arthritis considerably worse; and it kills people.

Obesity is often regarded as a social problem. I strongly suspect that most of the people who spend most of their lives dieting want to lose weight because they want to look better, to wear more fashionable clothes and to be more attractive to others. But even relatively mild obesity can produce or exacerbate high blood pressure, gout and diabetes. Heart disease occurs more frequently among people who are overweight. Hernias and skin problems are also common too. Here are some of the ways in which being overweight can affect your health:

Your skin

Fat people have deep skin creases which are difficult to keep clean and dry – so fungus infections are commonplace. Because fat acts as a sort of insulation – keeping the body warm – overweight people sweat a lot in hot weather. This makes their skin problems even worse. Women who are overweight often find that their abdominal skin creases and the areas around their groins and under their breasts are particularly likely to cause problems. Eczema and dermatitis commonly develop. Losing weight will mean that fat disappears, but if the skin has been stretched for a long period of time the skin fold may not disappear – when this happens, surgery may be needed.

Your joints

Because they have more weight to carry around, fat people are far more likely to suffer from arthritis and rheumatism. Joints and ligaments simply begin to creak under the weight they have to carry. The knees are often the first to give way. Losing weight will not repair damaged joints, but it will dramatically reduce the incidence and significance of future problems. If you're overweight and you suffer from arthritis, then losing weight will usually mean that you'll suffer less pain and be more mobile.

Your heart

The heart has the job of supplying the rest of your body with fresh blood – delivering oxygen and taking away waste products. The more body there is, the harder your heart has to work. An average heart beats seventy times a minute. That's 4200 times an hour; 100,800 times a day; 705,600 times a week; 36,691,200 times a year and a staggering 2,568,384,000 times in an average lifetime. If your heart has to work 20 per cent harder (because you're 20 per cent overweight), the strain will eventually tell. A 1000cc engine may drive a small car very well, but put the same engine into a bus and there will soon be signs of strain. If you can lose your excess weight, then the strain on your heart will be reduced as will the risk of your suffering from heart trouble.

Your blood pressure

Normally, blood travels around your body under pressure – like water travelling through a hosepipe or through the pipes of a house. If you use a longer garden hose, you'll need more water pressure; if your body gets bigger, the blood pressure will have to increase. Inevitably, therefore, people who are overweight usually have high blood pressure. The danger is that a blood vessel will be unable to take the strain and will burst. That is often what happens when people have strokes. Lose weight and blood pressure falls – and you're less likely to have a stroke.

Your lungs

When you are at rest it may not be immediately obvious, but your chest is permanently expanding and contracting as air is sucked into and forced out of your lungs. When the chest wall is thick with fat respiratory movements become more difficult. This becomes noticeable even on slight exertion, when overweight people are likely to be short of breath. The shortage of fresh air in the lungs means a shortage of fresh oxygen in the blood – and that means that the heart has to work even harder to keep the tissues supplied. All this means that people who are overweight are not only more likely to suffer from heart disease but are also more likely to suffer from lung disorders such as asthma and bronchitis. Losing weight 'frees' the lungs and reduces all these hazards.

Your veins

Normally, blood in your legs gets back up to your heart through your veins. It is the muscles in your legs which help to squeeze the blood back upwards. In overweight people the muscles have difficulty in squeezing the veins, so blood stays there – producing swollen varicosities. Losing weight helps prevent this problem getting worse.

Those are just a few of the ways in which being overweight can affect your physical health. There are also many specific disorders known to be more common among people who are overweight.

For example, overweight people are far more likely to get diabetes than people of average or below average weight. Diabetes is caused by a malfunction in the pancreatic gland – the gland that produces the hormone insulin. Insulin helps the body make use of carbohydrates. Many people who develop diabetes – particularly those who develop the disease in adulthood – can eliminate all signs and symptoms simply by dieting and losing weight.

People who are overweight are also far more likely to develop gall bladder disease and hernias. They have more difficulty if they become pregnant, and they face extra risks if they need to undergo surgery as having an anaesthetic is far more dangerous if you are overweight.

HEIGHT-WEIGHT CHART *(MEN)*

Instructions for weighing yourself

1 Weigh yourself with as few clothes as possible and no shoes.
2 Measure your height in bare or stockinged feet.
3 You are overweight if your weight falls above your ideal weight band. You are underweight if your weight falls below your ideal weight band.

Height (feet & inches)	Metres	Ideal weight band (stones & lb)	Kilograms	Average weight (stones & lb)	Kilograms
5.0	1.52	8.5–9.5	53–59	8.12	56
5.1	1.55	8.6–9.6	54–60	8.13	57
5.2	1.57	8.7–9.7	54–60	9.0	57
5.3	1.6	8.8–9.8	54–61	9.1	58
5.4	1.62	8.11–9.11	56–62	9.4	59
5.5	1.65	9.2–10.2	58–64	9.9	61
5.6	1.68	9.6–10.6	60–66	9.13	63
5.7	1.7	9.10–10.10	62–68	10.3	65
5.8	1.73	10.0–11.0	64–70	10.7	67
5.9	1.75	10.4–11.4	65–72	10.11	68
5.10	1.78	10.8–11.8	67–73	11.1	70
5.11	1.8	10.12–11.12	70–75	11.5	72
6.0	1.83	11.2–12.2	71–77	11.9	74
6.1	1.85	11.6–12.6	73–79	11.13	76
6.2	1.88	11.10–12.10	74–81	12.3	78
6.3	1.9	12.0–13.0	76–83	12.7	79
6.4	1.93	12.4–13.4	78–84	12.11	81
6.5	1.96	12.8–13.8	80–86	13.1	83
6.6	1.98	13.0–14.0	83–89	13.7	86

HEIGHT-WEIGHT CHART *(WOMEN)*

Instructions for weighing yourself

1   Weigh yourself with as few clothes as possible and no shoes.
2   Measure your height in bare or stockinged feet.
3   You are overweight if your weight falls above your ideal weight band. You are underweight if your weight falls below your ideal weight band.

Height (feet & inches)	Metres	Ideal weight band (stones & lb)	Kilograms	Average weight (stones & lb)	Kilograms
4.10	1.47	7.5–8.5	47–53	7.12	50
4.11	1.5	7.7–8.7	48–54	8.0	51
5.0	1.52	7.9–8.9	49–55	8.2	52
5.1	1.55	7.11–8.11	49–56	8.4	53
5.2	1.57	8.1–9.1	51–58	8.8	54
5.3	1.6	8.4–9.4	53–59	8.11	56
5.4	1.62	8.6–9.6	54–60	8.13	57
5.5	1.65	8.10–9.10	55–62	9.3	59
5.6	1.68	9.0–10.0	57–64	9.7	60
5.7	1.7	9.3–10.3	59–65	9.10	62
5.8	1.73	9.7–10.7	60–67	10.0	64
5.9	1.75	9.10–10.10	62–68	10.3	65
5.10	1.78	10.0–11.0	64–70	10.7	67
5.11	1.8	10.3–11.3	65–71	10.10	68
6.0	1.83	10.7–11.7	67–73	11.0	70
6.1	1.85	10.9–11.9	68–74	11.2	71
6.2	1.88	10.12–11.12	70–75	11.5	72
6.3	1.9	11.2–12.2	71–77	11.9	74
6.4	1.93	11.5–12.5	72–78	11.12	75
6.5	1.96	11.8–12.8	73–80	12.1	77
6.6	1.98	12.0–13.0	76–83	12.7	79

Losing weight will help your body in a thousand ways. Even your feet will benefit! An average-sized pair of feet provide their owner with less than 50 square inches of support. Try supporting a bag of flour on the tip of one finger and you'll get an idea of the sort of strain I'm talking about. Losing weight will dramatically reduce the pressure on your feet and make bunions, corns and other similar problems far less likely.

How can you tell how much weight you need to lose?

Weight in relation to height

The simplest and most reliable way to see whether or not you are overweight is to weigh yourself. Unfortunately, many height-weight charts are useless. Some were devised over half a century ago when men and women were far less muscular than they are today – as a result, some of them indicate that *everyone* needs to lose weight!

And before you can use some height-weight charts you have to decide whether you have large, small or medium-sized bones! Apart from the fact that most people find this virtually impossible to do (how on earth can you really tell how big your bones are without first stripping off all the flesh?) there really isn't much point to the exercise anyway, since bones weigh relatively little and the differences between large and small bones are fairly small.

To help you judge your weight more accurately I've devised special height-weight tables which enable you to compare your weight with the average for your height and with the ideal weight band for your height.

If you weigh more than the average for your height then you are a little overweight, but if your weight falls outside the ideal weight band then your problem is more serious.

However, the height-weight charts aren't the *only* way that you can see how much weight you need to lose. Here are a few more techniques you can use to see just how much unwanted fat your body is carrying.

The pinch test

When medical scientists measure fat they use specially designed calipers. But if you want to find out just how much fat you're carrying all you need is your own fingers. Just pick up a lump of flesh between your thumb and forefinger and see how much space it takes up. Try this test on the back of your hand and you'll see that there isn't much fat stored there – but try the same test around your waist and it may be a rather different story. That's the first lesson. Fat deposits vary from site to site around your body.

The flesh you've picked up will contain two layers of skin and two layers of fat – and since human skin is fairly thin you've effectively got hold of two thicknesses of body fat. So to get an idea of the thickness of your body fat at that particular site you just halve the distance between your thumb and your forefinger.

With a little sleight of hand you can do this measuring yourself. But to begin with you may find it easier to measure with a friend. Don't squeeze until it hurts – just make sure that you have a firm hold. Then, using a ruler (it's probably easier to handle than a tape measure) measure the distance between the skin of your thumb and the skin of your forefinger.

The beauty of this test is that you can do it just about anywhere you can reach. However, the best place for the 'pinch test' is probably the triceps muscle at the back of your upper arm. You can also try measuring the body fat at your waist, on the back of your legs, on your thighs, hips and buttocks.

If the thickness of your skin and under-skin fat exceeds half an inch, then you've got too much fat there. And since the 'pinch test' measures a double thickness of skin and fat this means that anything more than one inch thick means too much fat.

The mirror test

This is perhaps the cruellest test of all. Stand naked in front of a full-length mirror. One good look will tell you *exactly* how much excess fat you're carrying – and where you're carrying it.

The tape measure test

Measure your chest and your waist with a tape measure. If your waist measurement exceeds that of your chest then you're carrying too much fat around your waist.

The ruler test

Lie flat on your back with no clothes on. Then rest a twelve-inch ruler on the bottom edge of your ribcage and the top end of your pelvis. If the ruler lies firmly on bone (with no flesh touching it in the middle) then you don't have a fat tummy. If the ruler bobs about, you probably need to lose weight from your waist.

Diets that don't work

The slimming business is constantly growing. It is already the biggest and most profitable part of the health care industry.

Theoretically losing weight is simple and straightforward. If you weigh too much it's because you've been taking in more food than your body has been burning up as energy. Your body only stores fat when you eat more than your body needs.

Traditionally, people who wanted to lose weight were encouraged to measure out their food intake and to make sure that they limited their calorie intake. By looking at calorie tables which list the potential energy content of different foods it is possible to match your potential energy intake to your projected energy output. The trouble with calorie counting is that it is tedious and boring. And since it encourages slimmers to become obsessive about their food it can be counter-productive. Many slimmers have ended up unable to think about anything other than food. To side-step these problems the slimming industry has offered would-be slimmers a wide variety of options. Here are some of the best-known – together with the reasons why they don't work.

The one-food miracle diet

New dieting theories come and go as regularly and as predictably as the seasons. During the last few years I have seen numerous slimming diets which have relied upon the supposedly miraculous properties of one particular type of food. The four most successful 'one-food' diets have involved eggs, apples, grapefruit and pineapples.

The proponents of the egg diet argued that eggs contain a mysterious enzyme which burns up other types of food so quickly that no fat can be stored. The advocates of the apple diet claimed that apples can detoxify and purify the human body – and can help slimmers achieve the weight they want rapidly and easily. The believers in the grapefruit diet said that grapefruit contain special fat-burning enzymes. They argued that the more grapefruit you ate the thinner you'd get. Theoretically, if you ate too many grapefruit you could disappear altogether. Finally, the backers of the pineapple diet claimed that *their* favourite fruit contained magical ingredients designed to turn any diet into a success story.

Sadly, there has never been a scrap of evidence to substantiate any of these wonderful-sounding theories. There is *no* magic food that slimmers can eat to burn up food or fat supplies.

The patented slimming pills

The advertisements are bold and unabashed. The claims are simple but dramatic. People buy these products – usually through the post – because they believe that they will be able to lose weight safely and painlessly, without any effort. The pills are often expensive but never worth buying. Most of them fall into one of three categories.

First, there are the pills which contain a laxative. By making your bowels function more frequently than normal these pills may cause a short-term weight loss. Invariably, however, the weight will return once the pills are discontinued. The main snag with these pills is that once you stop them you're likely to suffer from constipation.

Second, there are the pills which contain a diuretic – a substance which encourages a massive fluid loss. These pills are potentially dangerous because restricting the body's fluid content can seriously damage your kidneys. And the pills are quite useless because the moment you start drinking again you'll put weight back on again.

Third, there are the pills which fill your stomach so that you don't feel like eating. Once again the problem with these pills is that once you stop them you'll put back on any weight you've lost.

The prescribed slimming pills

There are several slimming pills now available which have to be prescribed by a doctor. Some of them work. Unfortunately, however, the most effective pills either contain or are related to a group of drugs known as the amphetamines, which are extremely addictive. Many would-be slimmers have become hooked on these pills, and so today no reputable doctor will prescribe them for any patient wanting to slim. The long-term disadvantages far outweigh any short-term advantages which may exist.

The low-fat diet

This diet involves cutting out all fat – including fat meat, all dairy products and any other foods which contain fat. Although, as I have already explained, fat can be a killer, I don't think that a long-term low-fat diet is a wise solution to a weight problem. Cutting out all fats is not the way to slim sensibly and effectively. The trouble is that we all need a proportion of fat in our diets. Without fat our skin becomes dry and our hair unhealthy. If you stayed on a low-fat diet for too long you could become deficient in vitamins A and D, which are both fat-soluble. There is also a danger that without any fat in your diet you could develop a serious mental disorder.

The high-fat diet

I really don't understand why, but the high-fat diet becomes popular and fashionable quite regularly. The aim is to eat masses of fried food, butter, cheese, milk and meat fat. This is, in my view, a nasty and dangerous way to diet. A high-fat regime usually causes diarrhoea, and although you will certainly lose weight temporarily because of this you will also lose fluids, vitamins and minerals. The consequences could be very dangerous. The other very real hazard is that a continual high fat intake may increase your risk of developing heart disease.

The low-carbohydrate diet

Once again, this is a dietary technique which I cannot recommend. Everyone needs *some* carbohydrates. This diet could easily lead to faintness, tiredness, irritability and dizziness.

The high-carbohydrate diet

The theory is that by eating plenty of cake, bread, biscuits, sugar and potatoes you'll be able to lose weight. As I've already explained, *some* carbohydrates are essential (and most of us do need to eat more of them), but a high-carbohydrate diet makes no real sense.

The low-fluid diet

If you follow this plan you can eat what you like — as long as you cut down on your fluid intake. I think this diet is dangerous and ineffective. Of course you will lose weight through simple dehydration. But you will have to start drinking again some time (or else you'll die), and the moment you do so you'll put the weight back on again. The low-fluid diet can never offer anything more than a temporary weight loss. It is also dangerous, since it will undoubtedly put a high strain on the kidneys.

The low-protein diet

To achieve a noticeable weight loss you would have to cut down your protein intake to a perilously low level. Your body would eventually start to break down its own protein stores — and that would mean that muscles would disappear. There is no guarantee that your heart muscle wouldn't be the first to suffer. A low-protein diet could lead to an early death.

The high-protein diet

This is another potentially hazardous way of losing weight. Anyone with a poorly functioning kidney or a kidney infection could easily put their kidneys under too much pressure — with disastrous results. To minimize the risk of kidney failure you would need to drink vast quantities of water every day. The additional fluid would probably lead to a weight gain!

Surgical miracles

Today a number of surgeons offer special operations to people who can't lose weight. The operations most commonly performed include:

- Jaw wiring – steel wire is used to bind the upper and lower jaws together so that no food can be swallowed. This technique is now known to be quite useless. Once the wires are removed any weight loss will be quickly regained.
- Stomach stapling – using staples to make the stomach smaller means that people can't eat as much at one sitting. But if you eat slowly it's easy to get around this technique.
- Balloons in the stomach – the idea is to make people feel full before they eat. But research has shown that this technique just doesn't work. People with a weight problem don't always stop eating just because they aren't hungry.
- Intestinal butchery – some surgeons chop out a huge length of intestine so that foods which are swallowed pass through more rapidly. The problem with this technique is that patients often suffer permanent, severe diarrhoea – and since essential nutrients aren't absorbed, special supplements have to be given.
- Liposuction – in which fat is sucked out of the thighs with a tube and a piece of equipment rather like a vacuum cleaner. The fat collects in a jar and is thrown away. This technique is to sensible slimming what skateboards are to family motoring.

I don't believe any of these techniques are worth trying. Indeed they all involve some danger, and should be avoided by all sensible slimmers.

Exercise gadgets

Rowing machines, static bicycles, aerobics classes – those are just three of the exercise techniques that have been recommended to slimmers. It is perfectly true that exercise will help any slimmer lose weight. After all, we only ever gain unwanted weight because our food intake exceeds the amount of energy we burn up through exercise. But exercise burns up excess energy at a pitifully low rate. Most people with a weight problem have difficulty managing more than fifteen or thirty minutes of hard exercise in any twenty-four-hour period, and that just isn't enough. To lose an appreciable amount of weight you need to exercise for several hours at a time – every day.

Those are just a few of the techniques which have been recommended to slimmers. There have been many more – some even more bizarre. Recently, for example, I even saw a diet based entirely on junk food! There are countless diet foods available, and an apparently unending variety of therapists prepared to offer dieting advice. But the final, sad, unavoidable truth is that most dieting techniques are doomed to failure from the start; most slimmers will never get slim by following any one of the magical, miracle diets.

For too many slimmers, dieting follows an entirely predictable pattern. They set off with great determination. To begin with, it works. They eat nothing but pineapples. They stick to their rhubarb and sprouts diet. They spend twenty minutes every morning sitting on their exercise cycle. And they lose a little weight. The initial weight loss may even be quite dramatic. There is a feeling that this may be 'it' – the diet of a lifetime.

But then, a week or perhaps a month later, the resolve weakens. The regime becomes boring and unappealing. The diet is gradually forgotten and the missing pounds reappear. Failure is inevitable because, although there is an enormous industry selling dietary advice, dieting is not the answer if you have a weight problem. If you go on a diet, the best you can hope for is a temporary weight loss. Slimming diets are all designed for short-term use. You can't stay on a banana diet for ever. Diets are boring and will make you ill. Sooner or later they all have to be given up. And if you haven't changed your old, bad eating habits, then the moment your dietary regime becomes boring, tiring, painful or uncomfortable and you resume those old habits the pounds will come bouncing back.

The real tragedy is that anyone who has *ever* managed to lose weight temporarily by dieting could get slim and stay slim with no more effort! There are no mysterious rules which say that just because you've been overweight for twenty years you have to stay overweight for the rest of your life.

The truth is that the slimmer who repeatedly loses weight, regains it and then loses it again uses up far more willpower than she would need were she to lose weight once and remain slim ever afterwards. If you really want to lose weight permanently, you must begin with that intention. Ignore trick diets which will lead only to a temporary weight loss. Make up your mind that you're going to lose weight for good.

You must plan a permanent change in your eating habits. And you must begin with the intention of *changing* your weight rather than simply losing weight. If you really want to lose weight for ever, decide now that you're going to learn to 'eat green' – and to change your bad eating habits permanently. It'll be much easier than you imagine. If you've *ever* dieted successfully – even if just for a week – you'll find my programme easy to follow.

Excuses you shouldn't make

We all make excuses when things don't go well. It's only human nature to look for an outside explanation. When a cake fails to rise the cook will blame the oven or the telephone call which interrupted at a crucial moment. When a racing car driver fails to win a race he'll blame his tyres, his engine, his mechanics or the road surface. When a politician fails to win an election he'll blame the weather, the dirty tricks played by the opposition or the unfair publicity he's received. When an author's book doesn't sell he'll blame the publisher, the booksellers, the sales rep and the literary editors who ignored his masterpiece.

So it's hardly surprising that when a diet fails the average slimmer will look around for a good excuse. And there are plenty of them to choose from. The trouble is, of course, that excuses are usually fairly feeble. Here are some of the excuses slimmers most commonly make, together with my explanation as to why these excuses really don't work.

My partner likes me plump

I really can't remember how many times I've heard this excuse. It's wheeled out with monotonous regularity – and it really is beginning to squeak a little now. If you're tempted to use this excuse to salve your conscience after yet another failure, then ask yourself whether your partner likes you *because* you are plump, or *despite* the fact that you are plump! There is one simple trick that you can use to help demolish this excuse for ever. Take off all your clothes and stand in front of a full-length mirror. That is what your partner sees.

I've always been fat – there isn't anything I can do about it

I'm prepared to believe the first half of this excuse – but not the second half. It may well be true that you've always been fat, but that, I fear, is merely a sign that you've always eaten more food than your body needs. If you want to be slim, you can.

I've got big bones

So what? Bones weigh remarkably little. However big your bones may be, they don't explain rolls of fat. If your bones are huge then they may, just *may*, add another few pounds to your weight. That's all.

But food is my main joy – the only real fun I get out of life

Is that *really* true? If it is, then you need to look hard at your life. There's nothing at all wrong with enjoying your food, but food should only play a *part* in your life. Once food takes over completely, overweight isn't the only problem you're going to have to face.

I'm too busy to diet properly

You're kidding yourself. It doesn't take time to diet. You don't have to spend hours preparing slimming menus or weighing every portion of food that is destined to pass your lips. All you have to do is to make sure that you only ever eat when you are hungry – and that you stop eating as soon as your hunger has been satisfied. However busy you may be, you can still diet successfully and lose unwanted weight permanently. In fact, think about it logically: since eating takes time and you're busy, it stands to reason that if you spend less time eating then you'll have more time for the other things in your life.

Everyone in my family is fat

Probably because they all eat too much. It's true that overweight – or rather the tendency to overweight – is sometimes passed down in families, but it's also true that bad eating habits are passed down from one generation to another. You may not be able to change your height or eye colour, but you *can* change your weight.

I can't afford to diet

This excuse may have stood up well when you were thinking about attending aerobics classes and buying special packs of slimming food. But the *Eat Green* diet is going to be cheaper than your old diet. By not buying large quantities of meat you're actually going to *save* money!

Slimming is a sexist activity – I'm not prepared to be caught up in it

Over the last few years many authors have argued that women who deliberately try to lose weight are being manipulated by men. It's nonsense. This argument has more holes in it than a fishing net. A woman who slims will probably be more attractive to men, it is true. But she will also benefit enormously herself. She will be healthier. She will be able to have more fun. She'll be able to wear a wider range of clothes. And she'll probably live longer too. Is any of that sexist?

It's my age

I've heard this excuse put forward by a sixteen-year-old, a twenty-five-year-old, a thirty-four-year-old, a forty-two-year-old, a fifty-nine-year-old and a sixty-seven-year-old. It's about as accurate as a politician's promise.

I can't diet because I have to eat out a lot

Eating out has nothing to do with eating too much – or getting fat. Simply choose the least fattening item on the menu – and eat only what you need!

You may think that I'm cruel to 'destroy' all these well-established excuses. But I'm really trying to help. It won't help you diet successfully if I sympathize with you and allow you to continue to use your favourite excuse as a reason for failing. In the long run my sympathy won't help you at all.

If you're going to deal with your weight problem effectively and permanently, you have got to learn to forget about excuses. There will *always* be an excuse available. There will always be something or someone that you can blame for the fact they you are overweight – and your failure to lose your excess weight permanently. If you *sincerely* want to lose weight and stay slim, you have to find the courage to admit that you have a weight problem because your body hasn't needed the food you've eaten.

Don't let an addiction to food ruin your diet

Thousands of people who are overweight eat too much because they are addicted to food – not just any food (I'll deal with a general obsession with food on page 131) but specific types. Food can be as addictive as drugs, and your irresistible urge to eat could be the craving which is wrecking your diet. If you are hooked on food, then until you break that addiction your slimming efforts will be doomed to failure. There are two main types of food addiction – psychological and physical. I'll deal with the psychological form first because it's the simplest.

Psychological food addiction

To a very large extent our eating habits are created by circumstances. If, when you were small, your parents re-warded your good behaviour and good deeds by giving you food, then you will have grown up to associate particular types of food with praise and with feeling happy. Millions of people love eating sweet things because these are the types of food that parents most commonly give as a reward.

When a mother gives her child sweets because he has been 'good' or allows him to have his pudding only when he has eaten up all his vegetables, she is training him to associate food with behaviour and to learn bad eating habits that will probably last him a lifetime. Similarly, parents may instil a

---

hatred of certain foods by forcing children to eat them. For example, if your parents made you eat cabbage even though you didn't like it and didn't want to eat it, you will almost certainly still hate cabbage and associate it with unpleasantness, unhappiness and general misery. (Incidentally, if your parents had given you green vegetables as a reward and made you eat sweets as a punishment, you would now very probably love spinach and cabbage and hate eating anything sweet!)

QUESTION: *Isn't meat addictive? If I stop eating meat will I suffer withdrawal symptoms?*

ANSWER: *Meat can be habit-forming, and most people who give up meat do notice a slight craving for a few weeks afterwards. You may find that when eating out you'll look across at your non-vegetarian companion's plate with some envy. But these cravings disappear, and after a few months you will probably wonder how on earth you managed to eat anything so repulsive. I now find the smell of meat quite nauseating, and the sight of a steak or a bacon sandwich puts me off my food!*

This type of food addiction is produced by a process known as conditioning and it can be very difficult to break. It is, indeed, this sort of bad eating habit that is the cause of a great deal of obesity these days. We all have an appetite control centre in our brains and if, from childhood, we are allowed to eat what we want, when we want, and in the quantities we want, then by and large we do not put on excess weight. Experiments done with children have shown that the appetite control centre is quite capable of deciding for us what foods we should eat and when we should eat them. Unfortunately, the parental conditioning that most of us go through destroys that natural ability and leads us to confusion and distress.

Parental conditioning isn't the only active force, of course. We are also subjected to many other pressures. Women, in particular, are constantly under pressure to achieve the right shape and the right size. For most of the twentieth century the 'ideal' female shape as advocated by fashion designers and trumpeted by the fashion press has been slender and boyish.

This type of coercion, when accompanied by other social and parental influences, can eventually result in the development of conditions such as anorexia nervosa and bulimia nervosa. These are not addictions but disorders linked to our general attitude towards food.

One of the foods most commonly used for comfort eating is chocolate. Advertisers have for years taught us to associate chocolate with childhood and with happy times. So it is perhaps not surprising that addiction to chocolate is one of the commonest of all food addictions. But chocolate addiction is not just psychological – there is also a strong chemical or physiological element to this type of addiction.

Physiological food addiction

Over the last few years I've had countless letters from chocolate addicts. Inevitably, perhaps, they have all had a weight problem – chocolate is, after all, extremely fattening.

As I've already explained, many people get hooked on chocolate because it is the food which we most commonly learn to associate with feeling 'happy' and 'contented'. Look at chocolate advertisements and you'll see that they invariably support that association. The words 'chocolate' and 'love' are never all that far apart. So when we're feeling lonely, sad or bored we often buy chocolates to cheer ourselves up. Subconsciously we think we're buying love, affection and approval. But that's only the psychological aspect of chocolate addiction. There is also a chemical element to the addictive process.

This was first explained a few years ago by three experts working at New York's State Psychiatric Institute. They had discovered a natural substance in the brain called phenylethylamine, which is rather similar to the amphetamines. It is this chemical which in normal, healthy humans is responsible for the highs and lows of being in love. We feel good when we are in love because the amount of phenylethylamine in our brains is unusually high. The pleasure we experience is rather similar to that felt by an amphetamine user. When a love affair comes to an end we suffer the sort of low feeling that is common among amphetamine users when they stop taking their drugs. People get hooked on chocolate because it can even out the ups and downs of everyday life – and because it is readily available at a relatively low price.

Scientists used to think that chocolate was unique in being a food that can cause a genuine type of physical addiction. Today, however, scientists recognize that it is perfectly possible to get addicted to many other types of food. The ones which most commonly cause problems include corn, wheat, milk, eggs and potatoes, and the addiction these substances produce is similar in quality to the type of addiction produced by alcohol.

Not surprisingly, people who get hooked on particular types of food almost invariably end up with a weight problem. The strange thing is that, if you're suffering from this type of food addiction, it is almost certainly because you are allergic to the food that you're hooked on! If you feel there are one or two particular foods which you can't do without, there is a very good chance that your passion for them is hiding a powerful allergy reaction.

Scientists now know that it is possible to be allergic to a particular type of food in exactly the same way that a hay fever sufferer may be affected by pollen or a penicillin-sensitive patient may be allergic to that drug. The normal symptoms associated with a food allergy include lethargy, depression, exhaustion and irritability, but they can usually be hidden or suppressed by eating the food that causes the allergy! If that sounds difficult to believe, just remember that a patient can be protected against the symptoms of hay fever by giving him or her a series of injections which contain active ingredients from the pollen to which he or she is allergic!

Eating the food to which you're allergic disguises the symptoms very effectively, and the patient simply feels that he or she has a weak will and a strong craving for a particular type of food. Obviously, the richer in calories a food is, the more likely it is to produce a weight problem. If you're a wheat addict and you eat two extra slices of bread a day, in a year you'll put on an extra stone in weight!

Researchers in America have shown that people get hooked on food in much the same way that alcoholics get hooked on alcohol. Indeed, when a number of American alcoholics were studied it was found that they were allergic to corn, malt, wheat, rye, grapes and potatoes. It seems possible, therefore, that many alcoholics drink too much because they are allergic to the basic foods from which their favourite beverage is made.

How can you tell if you are a food addict?

Answer all the questions as carefully and as honestly as you can. If you answer 'Yes' to three or more questions, the chances are high that you are suffering from a food addiction. Your problem may have a psychological or a physiological basis.

1 Do you enjoy food very much?
2 Do you ever get cravings for particular types of food?
3 Do you frequently think – or even dream – about food?
4 Do you have any allergies – e.g. hay fever, eczema or drug allergies?
5 Are there any foods which you eat most days?
6 Do you ever feel happier, more content or physically more at ease after eating?
7 Do you get edgy or irritable if you go without food for long periods?
8 Do you ever need to get up at night and nibble?
9 Have you ever suffered from a food allergy in the past?
10 Do you ever suffer from a headache if you miss your favourite food for a few hours?

How to deal with a food addiction

If you are a food addict, you need to deal with your problem now – otherwise your attempts to diet will never prove successful. Here's how you can 'kick' your food addiction:

1 First you must identify the food to which you are addicted. It may already be obvious. If not, every food that you eat at least once every three days must fall under suspicion. Remove foods from your diet – one at a time – for seven days at a time. Then reintroduce each food one by one. If you are allergic to a food you will feel irritable when you go without it – and you will develop unpleasant symptoms (for example a headache) within a few hours of eating it again. I suggest you get your doctors help before doing this.

2 Once you have identified the food to which you are addicted, you may find it easier to cut down your consumption of it in easy stages. So, if you think you are a chocolate addict, cut down your consumption slowly over a period of one or two weeks – just as you would cut down on cigarettes if you were trying to stop smoking. If you're feeling braver, then you may be able to go 'cold turkey' and cut out chocolate completely overnight. But be warned! You may suffer unpleasant side-effects for a few days.

6

The Ten Super Secrets of Permanent Slimming Success

Over the last twenty years I have talked to thousands of slimmers – and exchanged letters with thousands more. I have learned that all slimmers face – and must overcome – the same basic problems if they are to succeed.

Here are the ten vital steps you must take if you are to diet successfully – with lasting success. Read the advice on the following pages carefully and you will be able to lose weight – and stay slim – without any calorie counting, without any painful exercises and without any boring, fixed menus.

Secret no. 1

Never forget *why* you want to lose weight

Many slimmers endure endless agonies: they weigh out every item of food; they count their calories; they perform difficult, painful and tedious exercises; and they spend a fortune on equipment and classes – but they never really have a clear idea of just what they're going to gain by being slim. If you don't know exactly how you're going to benefit by losing weight, you'll almost certainly fail. To slim successfully, you have to sort out what the advantages are going to be so that you are properly motivated. Don't let your diet fail for lack of motivation. Here are just a few of the benefits you'll enjoy if you lose unwanted weight:

● you will be healthier

- you will be able to wear more exciting clothes – and you'll probably be able to buy bargains in the sales, too
- you'll have far more confidence
- you'll be able to enjoy sports and social occasions much more

You can probably think of another dozen advantages. So do just that – think of the ways in which your life will be better when you've lost weight. Then write down your reasons and keep your list somewhere close at hand – so that you can look at it several times a day. Remember: if you sincerely, genuinely and honestly want to be slim, you will succeed.

Secret no. 2

Start a compost heap

Do you dislike throwing food away? Do you find it difficult to put down your knife and fork when there is still food left on your plate? If, when you are clearing plates away from the table you see perfectly good food left over, do you ever eat any of it? Do you ever eat up the crumbs in the biscuit tin?

When I conducted a survey of slimmers I found that over half of all people with a weight problem admitted that they felt terribly guilty if they ever had to throw food away. Just under half admitted that they would always eat food rather than throw it away, and a third rather shamefacedly admitted that they frequently ate other peoples leftovers.

This cautious, respectful attitude towards food is something that most of us acquire when we are young. We are encouraged to eat up all the food on our plates by mothers who frequently remind us that there are starving people who would be grateful for the food we don't want to eat. Consequently we grow up feeling guilty whenever we leave anything on our plates or throw food away. We will (albeit with some pangs of guilt) throw out clothes that are worn out or grossly unfashionable, but too often we find that we just cannot throw food away. I've known slimmers who would rather put a piece of mouldy cheese into their mouths than throw it into the dustbin. I've known slimmers who would eat food they didn't even like rather than throw it away.

It's daft, isn't it? Your body doesn't need the calories. And all that food is merely going to be stored as fat. You're probably going to have to spend weeks losing those pounds that you should never have gained in the first place. The fact is, of course, that you aren't helping anyone by using your stomach as a dustbin and eating unwanted leftovers. No one in Africa or India will eat any better because you aren't throwing food away. You aren't saving any lives by eating up those leftovers. In fact, by perpetuating bad habits you are harming your health. When you pass on those bad habits to others (for example your children) you are simply creating new problems – not solving any old ones.

I realize that learning to throw out food can be difficult; the old, long-established barriers of guilt can be difficult to break down. The only way to succeed is to practise. Try it now. Go into the kitchen and look through the cupboards and the fridge. Then throw out unwanted or stale bits of food. Throw out stuff that you know you aren't ever going to use. If you have a garden, start a compost heap – knowing that the food you're throwing out is being used will probably make you feel better.

Finally, here are a few extra tips that will prove helpful:

- Try to be more accurate when guessing how much food people will eat. Most cooks prepare too much rather than too little, particularly when entertaining guests.
- If you always seem to prepare too much food, don't put everything you prepare on to the table. Leave some in the kitchen. If it's needed, you can bring it out; if it isn't needed, you can always put it in the fridge or freezer to be used another day.
- Make a collection of recipes suitable for leftovers. You won't feel so bad about having food uneaten if you know that you can use it up afterwards.
- Have a supply of small, sealable containers ready for storing leftovers.
- Remember that 'green' food is much easier to store than meat. And your compost heap will always welcome 'green' leftovers!

Secret no. 3

Don't eat in the evening

I've lost count of the number of slimmers I've met whose main problem has been night-time nibbling. During the daytime they hardly eat at all – but in the evenings, while sitting down watching television, they hardly ever stop! And most of the food they eat is, of course, extremely fattening: biscuits, crisps, peanuts and chocolates. Night-time nibbling has nothing to do with hunger but is usually done to allay boredom. The nibbler doesn't stop when he or she is no longer hungry, because hunger has nothing to do with it.

The main problem with eating during the evening is that most of the food which is consumed isn't needed – and so it is stored as fat. Some slimmers believe that it doesn't matter *when* you eat as long as you limit your intake of calories. But this simply isn't true. Calories consumed at night are far more deadly than calories consumed in the morning.

When you eat five hundred calories at breakfast-time they will be converted into blood sugar within a relatively short time. And since the chances are high that you'll be busy early in the morning, your body will burn up that sugar to satisfy its immediate energy needs.

However, when you eat a meal of five hundred calories at supper-time the consequences are rather different. Once again the calories will be converted into blood sugar, but this time your body won't have any immediate need for them. Your body burns up far fewer calories when you are slumped in front of the television set or lying in bed than it does when you are rushing around doing the shopping and the washing or getting to work. So in order to prevent your blood sugar levels rising to intolerable – and even dangerous – levels much of that unused potential energy is converted into fat, to be stored for future use.

By the time you wake up the following morning – and start to get yourself ready for the day ahead – your blood sugar will be relatively low again. And as you rush around you will feel uncomfortably hungry. Your body will need energy supplies quite quickly. In theory you don't need to respond to that feeling of hunger because your body has stored plenty of calories from the food you ate the night before. And if you ignore the rumblings in your tummy and the slightly light-headed feeling that you have, all will be well. Your body will obtain the energy supplies it needs from the calories you ate yesterday evening.

But, in practice, that isn't likely to happen. You'll eat more food – and obtain the energy you need from a fresh supply of calories. Inevitably, your attempts at dieting will be in tatters and you will put on weight. The calories which you ate during the evening, and which were stored for some future use, will stay stored.

Here are some tips designed to help you control night-time nibbling more effectively:

- Stop buying high-calorie fattening nibbles. Make sure that if you *do* nibble you nibble slimming biscuits or sip at low-calorie drinks. Keep apples, bananas or oranges handy – rather than packets of biscuits or roasted peanuts.

- Try to keep yourself busier during the evenings. One of the reasons why most people find it easier to avoid nibbling during the daytime is that they are busy with other things and don't have too much time to think about food or succumb to the temptation to nibble. Try to get out of the house more in the evenings. Perhaps you could enrol in a night school course. Perhaps there are clubs or groups which you could join. Maybe you could take up a sport or a hobby to which you could devote more attention. If you spend long periods of time watching television, take up knitting or embroidery or crocheting – all will keep your fingers busy and away from the biscuit tin.

- If you're trying to break bad eating habits, move all the furniture round in your living room. When you sit down to watch the television sit in a different chair – or move your favourite chair to a new position. Change the easy things – and you'll find bad habits easier to break (that's why switching to a 'green' diet is going to make dieting easy for you).

- Buy vegetarian nibbles rather than sweets and chocolates. Nuts, dried fruit and raisins aren't particularly low in calories, but you're less likely to get hooked and eat your way through a whole boxful of calories! Besides, you can take some small comfort from the fact that vegetarian nibbles are at least packed with goodness.

Secret no. 4

Only eat when you're hungry

It is now over half a century since one of the most remarkable research projects ever planned was first described in an American medical journal. Until I unearthed the scientific paper that described the research work, it and its astonishing conclusions had been forgotten. And yet that one experiment provided the basis for all sensible slimming programmes.

It led the way to the discovery of the appetite control centre – an impressive, automatic device hidden deep inside every human brain. The power of this unique control centre is quite astonishing: it can make sure that you never get underweight or overweight, and that you never become short of essential vitamins or minerals.

The experiment was performed by Dr Clara M. Davis of Chicago in the 1920's, and she first published her results in the *American Journal of Diseases of Children* in October 1928. Dr Davis had three aims. She wanted to know whether the young, newly weaned infants she had chosen for her experiment could:

1 Choose their own food and eat enough to stay alive.
2 Select a good balanced diet without any outside help.
3 Pick foods which would help them to stay healthy.

The results were staggering. Dr Davis found that without any prompting the infants automatically chose good, varied diets. Their growth rates, development, vigour and appearance were just as satisfactory as those of babies who had been eating foods carefully selected by expert dieticians and nutritionists. The young children ate the right types of food in the right amounts, and they stayed healthy.

Five years later Dr Davis produced details of more research work that she had done. Having studied fifteen infants for between six months and four and a half years, she had come to the conclusion that they were all able to select a good variety of satisfying foods and to ensure that they ate neither too much nor too little. Despite the fact that none of the children had been told what to eat, they all remained healthy. Their eating habits seemed to be unplanned, even chaotic, but none of them ever suffered from stomach ache or became constipated. None of the children who was allowed to choose his or her own food became fat or even chubby.

Some years later, during the Second World War, a larger and more sophisticated experiment, organized by army doctors, showed that when soldiers are allowed access to unlimited supplies of food they eat what their bodies need according to the environment. Without any professional prompting or guidance, the soldiers automatically chose a mixture of protein, fat and carbohydrate that was appropriate for their immediate needs.

The only conclusion to be drawn from these experiments is that if you listen to your body – and eat when it tells you to – you will not go far wrong. If, in addition, you can make sure that you eat the foods your body tells you to eat and that you stop eating when your body tells you to stop, you'll not only stay healthy but you'll also stay slim.

I've explained the importance of the appetite control centre to numerous slimmers over the last few years. And everyone who has learned to use it has gained enormously in confidence and in slimming success. As far as I know there has never been a failure. Everyone who has used the techniques I've devised, which are based on the existence of this control centre, has successfully lost weight – and, even more important, stayed slim.

But to start with, just about everyone has been sceptical. 'If there is such a marvellous device in my brain,' they say, 'then why am I fat?'

The answer is simple. Most of us have lost the art of listening to our own bodies, and we've acquired many bad eating habits which over-rule out internal appetite control centre. We no longer eat simply because we are hungry – we eat for all sorts of other reasons too. Boredom, guilt and depression are probably the three most dangerous enemies of any slimmer. Thousands and thousands of women and men regularly eat not because they are hungry or because they *need* food but because they are bored, feel guilty or are depressed.

Boredom is one of the commonest and yet one of the most under-estimated problems in society these days. It affects millions: people who have dull, routine, uninspiring jobs; people who have retired early; and people who have no job at all. In a special survey I conducted recently, I discovered that 87 per cent of people with a weight problem admitted that they regularly ate to cheer themselves up, while 91 per cent of slimmers admitted that they regularly ate because they were bored. Can you honestly say that you've never munched a biscuit for no other reason than that you were bored?

The only answer, of course, is to try to add more excitement to your life. Start going to evening or day classes at a local college. Take up a hobby that you find fascinating and rewarding. Begin a small business of your own at home. None of these activities need cost you much money – just time and a little effort. If you give yourself something to think about, and something to keep your mind occupied, the chances are that you won't get bored so often. And you won't end up trying to relieve your boredom by eating.

Guilt is underestimated as a driving force, too. Many slimmers don't have to do anything to feel guilty. They feel guilty simply because they are overweight. They feel that they are letting themselves or their partners down. They feel guilty for ever having put on so much weight. And they feel guilty for having failed to get the weight off again. As soon as they eat something fattening, even more guilt piles on. All that guilt then produces depression and shame, and the depression and shame lead directly to misery and unhappiness. Too often more food is seen as the answer.

We learn to associate food with our emotions when we are small, as I described earlier when talking about psychological food addiction. Gradually, over the years, we get into the habit of associating happiness with food – particularly sweets and other fattening food. The only way you can break this link is by learning to cheer yourself up in other, less fattening ways. Pick up the telephone and talk to a friend if you feel like breaking into the biscuit tin. Do some vigorous vacuuming or go out for a brisk walk if you're feeling miserable and are tempted to start comfort eating. Buy yourself a new book, magazine, record or tape if you feel glum. Get yourself a bunch of flowers or a new jumper.

Over the years thousands of women have admitted to me that they have a weight problem because they have allowed their emotions to dictate their eating habits. I can still remember the first time I ever spoke to a slimming group. I asked the women members of the class why they thought they had a weight problem. Amazingly, it was a question that none of them had ever tried to answer before. And even more amazingly, none of them could give me a serious reply. Everyone managed quick, easy, slick, traditional answers.

'I like food too much,' said a thirty-five-year-old housewife.

'I just can't say "No",' giggled a twenty-nine-year-old catering manageress.

'My hormones,' answered a forty-one-year-old mother of four, without really meaning it. None of them could *really* say why they had a weight problem, and yet they all desperately wanted to lose weight.

'Would you all agree that you weigh too much because you eat too much?' I asked them.

One by one they agreed that this comment was fair.

'So, to find out why you all have a weight problem we only have to find out why you eat too much?'

My slimming group agreed with me.

'When did your weight problem start?' I asked the housewife.

She thought carefully for a few moment. 'About a year after I got married,' she said at last.

'Your weight was stable before then?'

'It had gone up and down a bit, but it had never been too much of a problem,' she told me. 'It was after I got married that it really became a big problem.'

'Why?' I asked bluntly.

She said nothing for a full minute.

'Several reasons,' she said at last, very seriously. 'I had given up my job and I was bored at home. I started nibbling between meals. The usual things – chocolate biscuits, cake and so on. I also started having trouble with my mother-in-law. That upset me a lot and I got quite depressed.'

'So you started eating too much because you were bored and depressed?'

The housewife nodded.

'What about you?' I said, turning to the catering manageress.

'I've always had a weight problem,' she said firmly.

'Always?' I asked.

'Well, since I was about twelve or thirteen,' she replied.

'Can you remember why you started eating too much at that age?'

Once again it took quite a while for the full answer to emerge. But emerge it did.

'When I was twelve I had an enormous bust,' she said, blushing a little. 'I was ever so embarrassed by it. I went to a mixed school and the boys used to make awful comments. I used to cry every time I got home from school. My mum always tried to cheer me up by giving me lots of chocolates and stuff like that. After a while I found that the extra weight I'd put on meant that I didn't get so many rude remarks. My bust wasn't so prominent when I was fat all over, so the boys stopped making remarks.'

'And you've been fat ever since?'

She nodded.

'And you?' I said to the mother of four. 'Can you remember when your weight problem started?'

'It started after my first boy was born,' she told me. 'I was ever so depressed at the time, and then my husband had an affair with someone he worked with. If I wasn't screaming and shouting at him I was sobbing my heart out in the bedroom.' She paused for a moment. 'I ate to cheer myself up,' she admitted. 'It was as simple as that.'

I don't pretend that those three slimmers were typical. But they certainly weren't unusual. Over the years I've heard thousands and thousands of similar stories.

Every slimmer is different, of course. Everyone who develops a weight problem does so for very personal reasons. But in 99 cases out of 100, when someone develops a serious weight problem it is because they have been eating for all the wrong reasons – to cover up some sadness, or to help them cope with boredom. Clearly, therefore, one key to successful slimming must lie in learning to find other ways to deal with these very real problems, and in learning to regard food as a fuel rather than a comforter.

There are many reasons why people eat too much. Ask yourself the simple question I asked my group of slimmers: 'Why do you think you have a weight problem?' Try to think back to the days when you didn't have a weight problem. Then decide what changes influenced your eating habits. You may well be surprised by some of the answers you give yourself.

Next time you find yourself picking up a packet of biscuits or a piece of cake when you know you aren't really hungry, try to analyse the feelings which are uppermost in your mind. Try to decide exactly how you feel. Once you have worked out which emotional feelings are strongest when you start to over-eat, you'll be well on the way towards conquering your problem. Suddenly a lot of answers will become fairly clear to you.

You may, like many slimmers I've known, find that you eat too much when you're feeling lonely. If that's the case, it's clearly important to make some new friends and revive some of your old friendships. Join clubs and associations, write letters, ring people up. Find a part-time job or a post with a voluntary organization.

Once you've eradicated all your bad eating habits you can concentrate on learning to *listen* to your body when it talks to you. You can learn to eat only when you are hungry and to stop eating when you feel full. There is a simple but extremely effective trick you can employ here: every time you put food into your mouth ask yourself: 'Am I hungry? Do I need this?' After a while you'll find that your ability to listen to your body will improve; eventually your appetite control centre will regain its rightful authority over your eating habits.

Secret no. 5

Set yourself easy slimming targets

Nine out of ten slimmers set themselves impossible targets. When they decide to start losing weight they jump on the scales, work out how much weight they need to lose and aim to lose the lot in the first month. I have known slimmers who have expected to lose 40–50lb (18–22kg) in a matter of six or eight weeks. I've known slimmers who have been disappointed when they haven't been able to get rid of a lifetime's accumulated fat in a fortnight. A questionnaire I gave to slimmers showed that a massive 89 per cent were aiming at a target weight that was too low for them; nearly all these slimmers were hoping to lose their weight at an unrealistically rapid rate.

If you set yourself an impossible target (both in terms of the amount of weight you want to lose and in terms of the speed with which you lose it) then you'll fail. And when you fail you'll be depressed. You'll abandon your dieting plan. You'll return to your old eating habits. Failure begets failure.

So, begin by setting yourself a realistic target. Look at the height-weight tables on pages 100–101 and find out the average weight for your height. Then look at the acceptable weight band for your height. Then think about it carefully before you decide on the sort of weight you ought to be. Don't expect to be the same weight at forty as you were at sixteen. Don't aim at model-like slenderness if you've had three children. Be practical. Be realistic. Remember there is no point at all in setting yourself a target that you'll never be able to reach – let alone maintain.

Next, work out how much weight you need to lose in total. And then work out how long it's going to take to lose it. Work on a basis of losing 2lb (1kg) a week. That's a good, sensible, steady weight loss. If you lose weight at 2lb (1kg) a week then in three months you can lose 26lb (12kg), in six months you can lose 52lb (24kg) and in a year you can lose over 100lb (45kg)! If you lose more than 2lb (1kg) a week you'll probably get tired, weak and ill, endangering your physical and mental health and running a greater risk of failure.

Once you've worked out how much weight you need to lose – and how long it's going to take you to lose it – forget these figures and make yourself some short-term targets. Decide that in the next two weeks you're going to lose 4lb (2kg) and that in the next month you're going to lose 8lb (4kg). That's all you need to concentrate on. If you give yourself a small, realistic target then there is a great chance that you'll succeed. And if you succeed, you'll be a winner. You'll feel great. You'll feel like a successful slimmer. You'll feel good. Your confidence will get a boost and you'll tackle your *next* target with renewed enthusiasm and confidence.

Secret no. 6

Put food in its place

Ever since I first started writing about slimming I've received a steady stream of letters from people who have become obsessed both with food and with losing weight. Here's a typical letter:

Please help me. I am obsessed with food and dieting and it's making my life a misery. I feel really ashamed. I know I should be able to help myself, but I can't. From the moment I wake up I hardly think about anything but food. I just eat and eat and eat. In the morning I think about what I'm going to eat in the evening, and in the evening I think about what I'm going to eat the next day. I spend a lot of my time reading about diets and collecting magazine articles on slimming too. I'm overweight, I'm boring and I'm worried sick. Please can you help me?

This sort of obsession with food is extremely common – and nothing to be ashamed about. It's quite common for people who realize that they are overweight to put so much effort into losing excess pounds that they can think of virtually nothing else. They count calories, look for slimming foods, read diet books all day long and dedicate their lives to the search for slenderness. Eventually the obsession with dieting also becomes an obsession with food.

Of course, losing weight is important if you are overweight. I understand that well enough – I've met enough slimmers whose lives have been devastated by their excessive weight. But losing weight is not, and should never become, the *only* thing that matters in life. And it has to be kept in perspective.

The only way to beat this particular problem is not by concentrating on it (that will simply make things worse) but by doing exactly the opposite. Do your best to fill your life with so many other interests and enthusiasms that there just isn't time for your obsession with food to survive.

Begin by trying to define the other important things in your life. Make a list of all the people, ambitions and things which really mean something to you. Don't forget to include the simpler aspects of life. After people, we tend to think of homes, cars and clothes as being the chief things in our lives. They may well be. But there are many pleasures which won't cost you a penny to enjoy: lying on your back watching the clouds float by, having a cat sit on your lap, spending a warm day on the beach, walking in the soft summer rain, sitting by an old-fashioned log fire.

Try to put the other aspects of life into perspective. Try to remember what your ambitions were when you were a teenager. What did you hope to do with your life? Some things may be impossible now. But many of your dreams will still be attainable. You can still write a book, take up painting or learn to dance really well. You don't need much money to do any of these things – just time and patience. You can get all the books you need out of the public library, and find all the classes you need at your local adult education centre.

Think about work. Would you like to do something more satisfying? Do you want to try doing something else for a living? Are you prepared to start a new training course? Would you like to learn more about gardening or keeping animals? Would you like to take a car maintenance course?

It doesn't matter *what* you do as long as you start putting new things into your life. If you do, you'll benefit doubly. First, you'll enjoy the excitement and pleasure of a new occupation or hobby. Second, as you build up your other interests you won't find any time left for your pre-occupation with food.

The best way to beat an obsession is not to tackle it head-on but simply to put it in its place.

Secret no. 7

Build up your self-confidence

Confidence is very important in everything you do. If you pick up a pile of plates with confidence, you'll probably be able to carry them safely into the kitchen. If, however, you pick them up expecting to drop them, you probably will drop them. If you get on to a pair of skis and tell yourself you're bound to fall, then you'll fall. If you get into a motor car and tell yourself that you are going to have a crash, you probably will.

Likewise if you start a diet knowing in your heart that you're going to fail, then you'll almost certainly do so. A few months later you'll be worrying about your weight again — convinced that no diet in the world is ever going to work for you. Yet, amazingly, many would-be slimmers actually seem *proud* of their lack of confidence. Scores of letters come in to me from readers who say things like: 'I'm the world's worst slimmer', 'I'm no good at dieting' or 'You're not going to have any success with me.'

If you are going to lose weight permanently, you must have confidence in your ability to slim successfully. You must be able to say to yourself: 'I can do it. I can lose weight.' You must, in short, learn to have more confidence in *yourself*. There are several things you can do to build up your self-confidence.

1 If you lack confidence, the chances are that although you know very well what your weaknesses are you don't know what your strengths are. You are probably rather timid and shy (even though other people may not realize that), and you doubtless have little faith in your own abilities.

To counteract those fears sit yourself down with a piece of paper and a pencil and write down all the good things you can think to say about yourself. Everything. Imagine that you are writing an advertisement for yourself, and pick out all your very best points. You'll probably be amazed to see just how many virtues you have got. People who are shy and lack self-confidence tend to be unusually honest, generous, thoughtful and hard-working. You're probably exceptionally moral, careful, punctual, kind, ambitious and creative. List your physical as well as your mental attributes. If you've got lovely hair put that down. If you've got beautiful eyes or perfectly shaped feet, put them down. List everything good that you can say about yourself. Then, study your advertisement as often as you can in order to build up your own image of yourself.

2 Learn to put things into proportion. Many people who are slightly overweight regard themselves as being 'failures'. What

nonsense this is! Would you dismiss someone as worthless if there was one thing about them you didn't like or that wasn't perfect? Of course you wouldn't. Why, then, should other people regard you with contempt just because you happen to be overweight? Do you reject people as possible friends or business acquaintances just because they are skinny or bald or have small hands?

3 Don't be ashamed of your weight. If you have a weight problem, there are almost certainly some very good reasons for it. This book will have helped you discover what those reasons are. You can now set about solving your weight problem permanently. You should no more be ashamed of your weight than you are of your height or your hair colour. Until now you probably had no more control over your weight than you had over your height. Now that you *know* why you are overweight, you can deal with your problem speedily and successfully.

Once you have managed to change the way you feel about yourself you will, I think, find it much easier to deal with your weight problem. With more self-confidence and self-assurance you will be able to approach your weight problem from an entirely different angle. The more faith you have in yourself, the more successful your diet will be.

Secret no. 8

Stand up for yourself – be more selfish

I want to tell you about some patients of mine: first, a lady whom I will call Martha. When I met her she was really miserable. She was 6 stone (39kg) overweight and ashamed of it. She told me that one of her main problems was that, as a wife and mother of three children, she hardly ever stopped cooking.

'My husband gets cross if I don't eat with him,' she said. 'And the children are the same. They think there's something wrong if I don't sit down and eat when they have a meal.'

Martha's problem was that she was never, ever selfish. She never thought about herself or what she wanted. She was always too keen to please other people to be thinking about her own needs. She only managed to deal with her weight problem successfully when she broke free of her home and found herself a part-time job. Not being around at home all the time gave her a chance to run her own life a little more. And she soon found that she could stand up for herself.

Martha had forgotten how to think of herself as an individual. She'd forgotten that she had rights and needs. Her family were treating her as though she was a piece of kitchen equipment.

My second patient is a lady whom I'll call Teresa. Her problem was that she was too nice for her own good. When I first met her she was so anxious not to cause any offence that she was for ever being pushed around. She told me that her problem was Sunday lunch with her in-laws.

'They're very nice people,' she said, 'but my mother-in-law is one of those people who gets very offended if you don't have second helpings at every meal. I always end up eating far too much – even though I don't want it – and ruining my attempts at dieting. I've given up trying to lose weight now, because I know that all my effort during the week will be ruined on Sundays.'

Teresa, I soon found, was one of those kindly people who is always running errands for other people who can perfectly well do their own errands. She was the sort of person who always gets to look after all the children while everyone else goes off to the cinema or a party. I explained to her that she would only diet successfully when she changed her attitude and realized that she didn't have to be rude or aggressive to stick up for herself.

She wanted to know if I could suggest some excuses she could use when trying to refuse extra food that she didn't want, but I told her that excuses were no good.

'If you don't want more food, then you must say so – firmly but politely,' I told her. 'If you try to offer explanations or excuses, you'll probably end up trapping yourself and being manipulated into a corner. So, for instance,' I continued, 'if you try to avoid more food by saying that you're on a diet your hostess may disarm you with a compliment – telling you that you don't need to diet, that you look wonderful the way you are. If she does, the chances are that you'll be embarrassed, flattered and flustered – and before you know where you are you'll have another pile of food on your plate.'

I told Teresa that she had to say something simple and straightforward such as: 'I'm afraid I couldn't eat another morsel – but it was absolutely delicious.'

'But won't she think I'm being rude?' she asked.

'Would you think a guest rude if she said that to you?' I asked her.

'Of course not!' she replied.

'There's your answer,' I assured her. 'If someone pressures you even after you've said "No", then *they* are being rude – not you.'

Finally, I want to tell you about Belinda. She was in her twenties when I first met her – and she was very depressed.

She told me that after years of being overweight she had managed to lose a lot and get down to her ideal weight at the age of twenty-two. 'It took a lot of effort,' she said. 'But I was really determined and I managed it in the end.'

I looked at her, puzzled. She was clearly very overweight.

'I've put it all back on again,' she told me tearfully. 'It took me nine months to get it off and three months to put it back on again.'

She told me that she had been having lunch one day with her best friend, who had told her she was silly to have dieted. 'She said I looked skinny and unhealthy and that I was making myself ill and that I ought to start eating properly again,' said Belinda.

'What did you feel about that?' I asked her.

'I thought I looked really good,' said Belinda. 'I felt really happy with my weight. I felt healthier than I had done for years.'

'But?'

'But I allowed her to persuade me to have a huge meal when I only wanted a snack, and one thing led to another, and before I knew what was happening I'd put all the weight back on again.'

These three slimmers had one thing in common: they had all allowed themselves to be bullied and pushed into eating too much by other people. They all needed to assert themselves more.

This problem is a very common one. Every month I hear

---

from countless slimmers whose diets are being ruined because they don't like saying 'No'. They eat because they are worried about offending people. They accept food they don't really want so that they don't hurt other people's feelings. They find it difficult to refuse when the hostess pushes another piece of cake on to their plate. Their good intentions are ruined by their 'niceness'. When I asked a group of slimmers how often they found themselves eating food they didn't want because of pressure from other people, three-quarters said they would always eat everything they were given when having a meal with friends, and two-thirds said that they would accept unwanted second helpings too!

Most of the time people who have difficulty in saying 'No' confess to a fear that if they do say 'No' they will cause offence. But no real friend will be offended if you refuse food that you don't really want. And as I've already pointed out, you certainly don't have to be rude or aggressive when you refuse food.

If you suffer from this problem – and you have difficulty in saying 'No' with firm determination – practise refusing food in your mind. Imagine that you are at a dinner party and the hostess is trying to put another helping of pudding on to your plate. And imagine yourself saying 'No' quite firmly but politely. You can tell her that the food is delicious and that you've enjoyed it very much but that you really couldn't eat any more. The more you practise, the easier you'll find it when the problem becomes reality. Just remember: it isn't rude to say 'No', but it *is* rude to make people eat food that they really don't want!

Secret no. 9

Think yourself thin (and shapely)

You can never over-estimate – or under-estimate – the power of the human mind. Your chances of dieting successfully can be dramatically improved if you imagine yourself slim; if you imagine yourself the shape you've always wanted to be. Indeed, many experts would claim that the single most important factor which will decide whether or not you achieve the weight and shape you really want is your mental attitude.

I first became aware of the extraordinary power of the mind – and in particular of the imagination – when I read a report about something that had happened when the film *Lawrence of Arabia* came out in the sixties. The movie contained a number of long desert scenes in which Peter O'Toole, the star, was seen wandering around on the back of a camel. He was clearly hot, tired and thirsty. In just about every cinema where the film was shown, the managers noticed the same thing: sales of cold drinks and ice creams rocketed. The only possible conclusion was that the desert scenes had made the customers feel uncomfortably hot, and their bodies had responded to what they were seeing on the screen.

You can experience the influence of your imagination on your body next time there is a film on television or next time you rent a video from your local store. If the film you are watching contains lots of shots of explorers in the Antarctic huddled together in tiny tents, with icicles on their beards and their sleeping bags frozen solid, you'll probably hear the people who are watching with you complaining about the cold and reaching to turn up the fire. If the film is frightening, with lots of shots of dark passageways and creepy murderers, the people with you will be biting their fingernails, covering their eyes and rushing outside during the commercials to check that the back door is firmly locked and bolted.

Indeed, you probably don't need to watch a film to see your imagination at work; simply reading a good book should produce the same effect. If the story is sad the tears will start to pour down your cheeks. If the story is dramatic and you are worried about the safety of the hero then your heart will beat faster. If the story is frightening, the hairs will stand up on the back of your neck. In each case your body is responding not to reality (in the real world you may be lying in bed or in the bath) but to your imagination. You can prove the power of your imagination to yourself another way. Try putting a wooden plank on the floor. Then try walking along it. You'll almost certainly find it ridiculously easy. Now, try telling yourself that the plank is suspended hundred's of feet up in the air. And tell yourself that if you fall you will be dashed to death on the rocks below. Try to see the huge chasm beneath you.

Then try walking across the plank. The piece of wood won't have changed in width. And it will still be resting on the floor. But you'll find walking it a much more difficult task.

One of the first properly organised experiments designed to show the power of the human imagination took place some years ago. Researchers took a large group of people who had absolutely nothing in common apart from the fact that none of them had ever played basketball. After spending one day throwing basketballs through a hoop the volunteers were divided into three groups.

The first group were told not to play any basketball at all. They were told not even to think about basketball.

The people in the second group were told to practise every day for ten minutes.

The volunteers in the third group were told to spend ten minutes a day *imagining* that they were throwing balls into a basket.

At the end of one month the people in the first group were no better at basketball than they had been at the start of the exercise. However, the other two groups had improved by similar amounts. The players who had been spending their time out on the court physically throwing balls through hoops had improved by twenty four per cent. And the players who had spent ten minutes a day *imagining* that they had been throwing basketballs through hoops had improved by an amazing twenty three per cent.

Doctors have performed experiments to show what tremendous power the imagination can have over the body. For example, an American scientist told a number of volunteers to place their right hands in icy water and to hold them there for as long as they possibly could. If you think this sounds easy, just try it! After a few seconds, holding your hand in ice-cold water becomes a really painful experience. Your hand doesn't like it – and it will quickly let your brain know!

Then, for the second half of the experiment, the scientist told the volunteers to try and imagine pleasant scenes while their hands were in the icy water. They were told to pretend that instead of sitting in a laboratory they were in a beautiful, peaceful spot overlooking a wonderful, bright blue lake. They were told to imagine that it was a hot day and that the water was refreshingly cool. The results were very impressive. In the second experiment virtually all the volunteers managed to hold their hands in icy water for much longer than before.

Recently, doctors have harnessed the remarkable power of the human imagination in a variety of practical ways, for instance in helping patients overcome cancer. Migraine is one of the chronic, widespread problems now regularly treated with the aid of the imagination.

Migraine sufferers have to put up with headaches, nausea, mood changes, sensitivity to light and noise, itchy eyes, stuffed up noses and a host of other annoying symptoms. The headaches can be particularly severe and very difficult to treat. Although there are still some mysteries about precisely what happens during a migraine attack it seems that the problems are largely a result of the body's responses to stress. Misled into thinking that it can cope with the stress by preparing the muscles for immediate action, the body increases the blood supply to the muscles and closes down the supply to the brain. Then, when the threat seems to be lifting, the vessels open up again and the blood surges back through. It is this renewed flow of blood which seems to cause the pain of a migraine attack.

Many sufferers can ease the severity of their attacks by avoiding stress, by learning to cope with pressure more effectively, by not eating certain foods and by using drugs which interfere with the constriction of the blood vessels. But these techniques don't always work very well, and in the last year or two researchers have shown that it is perfectly possible to use the power of the imagination instead.

Stopping a migraine developing involves stopping the blood vessels constricting. But how? After all, you can't see or feel the arteries supplying your brain, so how can you possibly tell whether or not your efforts are working? Then someone noticed that migraine sufferers often have cold hands and cold feet, and someone else pointed out that when the blood vessels supplying the brain are constricted by the body's response to stress the vessels to the skin, hands and feet are also constricted. And that provided the clue!

For although it isn't possible to tell what you are achieving with the arteries that supply your brain, it *is* possible to tell whether or not your attempts to open up the vessels supplying your hands are successful. To defeat a migraine, therefore, a patient must make a conscious attempt to divert blood into the peripheral system which supplies the hands. If a patient can do this, and make his hands feel warmer, then he'll also be diverting blood into the vessels supplying his brain — thereby avoiding a migraine attack. However extraordinary all this may sound, the plain fact is that it works. Thousands of people now use this simple technique to control their otherwise uncontrollable pain.

The final experiment I want to tell you about is one of the most remarkable ever performed — and it proves without doubt the quite remarkable and far-reaching power that the mind can have over the body. It showed that simply by using their imaginations women could increase the size or shape of their breasts.

The technique depends on three facts. First, a woman's breasts swell and get larger when she is sexually aroused because of an increase in the flow of blood into the tissues. The increased blood flow is temporary, and so is the swelling of the breasts. Second, all the nutrients needed for tissue development are carried in the blood. If a part of the body has a good blood supply, then it will be healthy and grow larger than if it has a poor blood supply. Third, as I've already described, it is perfectly possible to increase the flow of blood to a particular part of the body simply by using the imagination.

The experiment produced emphatic and conclusive results. Women volunteers obtained a significant and lasting increase in breast size — 85 per cent confirmed that their breasts had definitely got bigger and nearly half had to buy bigger bras. There were other advantages, too — all the women reported that their breasts were firmer after using the technique, and volunteers whose breasts had become droopy and pendulous reported that the technique had improved the shape of their breasts.

I've described the power of the mind and the imagination at some length and included details of a few of the relevant experiments, because I believe these powers are important and I know that many readers will be sceptical. But I think that the evidence I've quoted shows conclusively that the human mind does have enormous power over the human body. The plain facts are that:

- if you start your diet really convinced that you are going to succeed, you'll stand a *much* better chance of succeeding
- if you start your diet telling yourself that you are going to have the shape you've always wanted, there is a very good chance that you'll succeed
- if you can close your eyes and 'see' yourself looking the way you want to look, you'll be helping yourself lose weight and get shapely

If you think positively the only thing you stand to lose is your excess weight. By using your imagination positively you will help yourself enormously. Finally, if you want to try using the power of your imagination for body shaping, read on.

The body shaping programme

Find somewhere quiet, where you can relax and be alone. Make sure that the curtains are drawn so that the room is dark and rather private. Take the telephone off the hook and put a 'do not disturb' notice on your door.

You must begin by regulating your breathing. Start by breathing in deeply. Count up to four while you are breathing in. Then hold your breath while counting up to two. Next, breathe out – again counting up to four as you do so. When you have emptied your lungs hold that position while you count up to two again – and then start the whole process again by taking another deep breath in. Breathing deeply will help to get your body and your mind into a gentle state of relaxation. Do remember that you must practise this technique regularly in order to obtain good results – twice a day for at least six months.

Next, relax your muscles one by one. Clench your left hand as tightly as you can – until the muscles of your hand and forearm feel tight and firm. If you then let your fist unfold you'll feel your muscles relax. Do this with every muscle in your body. Bend your left arm and try to make your biceps muscle stand out. Then relax and let the muscles loosen. Now turn your attention to your right hand and arm. When that is relaxed first tense and then relax the muscles of your feet and legs. Finally, relax the muscles of your chest, back, abdomen and face.

When your body is relaxed try to 'feel' yourself getting heavier and heavier. Try to 'feel' your body getting warm too.

When your body is completely relaxed you must relax your mind thoroughly. Imagine that you are walking along a quiet country lane. It is early summer and the lane is deserted. It is a beautiful, warm day. There is no traffic and you have no worries. The sky is a wonderful blue and the hedgerows are overgrown with colourful wild flowers. As you stroll along the lane you can hear the birds singing. You stand for a moment and look into a field. You can see poppies and many other wild flowers. Then you see a path on your right. Climb over a stile and follow the path along the edge of a field. It winds slowly down until it reaches a beautifully clear stream. The banks of the stream are quite steep and covered with soft, cool moss. You sit down for a moment, with your back resting against a tree, and look into the stream. You watch a kingfisher and two moorhens. Then you see a brown trout lazily swimming across to the opposite bank. You can feel the sun on your face, and the grassy bank and the tree make a wonderfully comfortable chair. You feel warm, happy, contented and relaxed. You have no worries, no anxieties and no fears. There is nothing you need to do and nowhere you have to go. You can feel your whole body absorbing the heat from the sun.

As you sit there on the edge of the stream you gradually become aware of your heart. You can feel it beating, slowly and regularly, deep inside you. Each time it beats, you can feel your heart pushing blood around your body. With your eyes closed you can 'see' that the blood vessels which supply the parts of your body which you want to shrink are getting smaller. You realize that your body is being redesigned, recontoured, reshaped, remoulded. Your body is being re-formed the way you want it.

You lie there for a few moments. You feel wonderfully calm and relaxed. You enjoy your private, personal place in the sun. You can feel the sun on your body. And you can feel your blood vessels deciding which parts of your body should get the best blood supplies. You can sense your body being reshaped the way you want it.

You realize that your body isn't going to change dramatically over night. But you're prepared to continue with the experiment. It is peaceful, restful and easy. You have faith. You believe that your body will soon be the way you've always wanted it. You feel confident and happy. You decide that you will repeat the experiment just as often as is necessary.

Secret no. 10

Give up eating meals

Most of us eat at fixed mealtimes. We eat at breakfast-time, in the middle of the day and again in the evening. This is, of course, a bizarre and thoroughly irrational way to behave. Our bodies don't just need injections of food three times a day – they need energy supplies all the time. By choosing to eat at standard mealtimes we make things difficult for ourselves in two ways.

First, for a host of different reasons we tend to eat too much when we sit down to a meal. We eat the food that has been prepared because we know that we are expected to eat it. We eat out of habit. We eat to keep other people company. And we eat whether or not we are hungry. Over the years we learn to eat according to the clock rather than according to our body's needs. Second, much of the food that we eat is, inevitably, not immediately needed. The energy sources are, therefore, converted into fat and stored for the future.

I think that all slimmers should attempt to abandon the idea of having three meals a day. There really isn't anything sacred about the idea of having three meals a day – it just fits in with the way that most of our lives are organized. Unless your life is planned in such a way that you *have* to eat three meals a day – at prearranged times – you're much better off eating whenever you happen to feel hungry.

If you feel a little peckish every couple of hours throughout the day, have a snack. Eating five or six or seven meals a day, rather than three large meals, will help your body adjust its calorie intake to its needs. People who have to eat at fixed times have to stock up with food so that they don't get hungry in between meals. If you snack, then you can afford to eat as much – or as little – as your body needs. You'll find it much, much easier to learn to listen to your body and to obey your internal appetite control centre.

Of course, you must remember that if you're allowing yourself to eat snacks throughout the day you can't have your three main meals as well. But you don't have to be unsociable and leave the family to eat alone. Give yourself less to eat, or just sit down with a cup of tea or one of your snacks.

You must also make sure that your larder and fridge are stocked with foods that you can use for snacking – otherwise you'll end up eating little but biscuits all day long, and you can't live on biscuits alone – they're pretty low in essential nutrients and pretty high in calories. So, buy the kind of food that will make it easy for you to create small, nutritious snacks whenever you happen to feel hungry. And then make sure that you prepare just enough to satisfy your appetite. Cut one slice of bread and make one half sandwich, for example. You can always make another sandwich afterwards if you're still really, genuinely hungry. If you open a can or a packet, don't think you've got to eat the lot just because its open. Prepare just enough to satisfy your immediate needs. Changing to the 'green' diet will help you change your eating habits from three meals a day to snacking when required.

Large meals are often meat-based. It's difficult to prepare meals that have meat in them without a lot of trouble, too. On the other hand, many vegetarian meals are very quick and easy to prepare and lend themselves very well to the snacking life.

Snacking really will help you enormously. There's plenty of evidence now available to show that people who nibble throughout the day, whenever they happen to feel hungry, will be far less likely to put on weight than those who stuff themselves with larger meals. By spreading your energy intake throughout the day you won't ever feel faint or hungry, and your body will learn to burn up all the calories you provide it with.

Remember: once food has been turned into fat it's difficult to get it turned back into potential energy. It's always much, much easier to turn food into fat than it is to turn fat into food!

7
The World's Best Slimming Tips

1 Every time you're about to put food into your mouth, ask yourself if you're *really* hungry.

2 If you feel hungry and find yourself reaching for food, try the five-minute delay tactic. Get the food ready if you like, but look at the clock and don't eat it for five minutes. Then, if you still feel hungry, eat it. If you have stopped feeling hungry put the food away.

3 Never eat just because it's time to eat. Most of us learn to eat at fixed mealtimes. Break away from this damaging habit. Eat when your body wants food – not when the clock wants you to eat.

4 Before you eat, decide what you want to eat. If you eat what you fancy, you'll probably leave the table satisfied. If you ignore what your body wants, the chances are that you'll leave the table unsatisfied – and eat more later. As I explained on page 124, our bodies are very good at deciding what we need to eat. Learn to trust your intuition.

5 If you're planning a big meal, have a small snack half an hour beforehand. A piece of fruit or raw vegetable, or a handful of raisins, nuts and dried fruit will do. The idea is to fill your stomach so that your appetite will be reduced.

6 Never eat standing up.

7 When you sit down to a meal, don't immediately start shovelling food into your mouth. Sit for a moment or two and relax. Try to get rid of any accumulated tensions. Look at the food in front of you. If you do this you'll be far more likely to hear your body 'talking' to you when it's eaten enough.

8 When you sit down to eat, don't talk, read or watch television. If you concentrate on what you're doing, you are

far more likely to hear your appetite control centre tell you when you're full.

9 At home, only ever eat in the kitchen or dining room. Don't allow yourself to wander around the house eating – or to take food into the living room, for example.

10 Turn the telephone off while you're eating. If you allow yourself to be interrupted, the chances are that you'll end up scoffing cold food quickly – and ignoring your appetite control centre.

11 Choose a small plate – if you eat from a big one there is a danger that you'll fill it and eat too much.

12 Always chew your food thoroughly! I know this sounds like an aphorism taken from the nursery, but it's worth remembering. If you chew food properly you'll have to eat slowly – and you'll be less likely to eat too much. But there's a bonus – you'll suffer less from digestive upsets.

13 Eat as many raw vegetables as you can – because they take a lot of chewing, they'll slow you down. If you eat slowly there is a much better chance of hearing your appetite control centre tell you that you're full.

14 Always put your knife and fork down between mouthfuls.

15 Stop between courses and rest. If you think you might have eaten enough, get up and walk around – maybe do something else. You can always return to the table for your next course if you still feel hungry.

16 If you eat Chinese or Japanese food use chopsticks – it's difficult to eat quickly when using chopsticks.

17 Learn to enjoy your food. Get into the habit of tasting each mouthful.

18 After you've finished a meal don't stay at the table if there is any food still on it. Many people who linger after a meal end up cutting themselves another piece of cheese or nibbling an extra biscuit – often without realizing. Leave the table as soon as you've finished eating – and clear away all the food.

19 Occasionally (and only occasionally) you can try sucking a toffee to appease your hunger and dull your appetite. If you're feeling peckish, pop one in your mouth. Your blood sugar level will rise and your hunger pangs will disappear.

20 Alternatively, try sucking a glucose sweet. Pharmacists now sell these for athletes since they help boost the blood sugar. An occasional one will help take away the hunger pangs and keep you going for another hour or two.

21 Don't spend money on special slimming products – you don't need them on the 'green' diet.

22 Don't worry about weighing your food. I've known many slimmers who've bought small scales and weighed every morsel of food they've prepared – and then worked out the calorie content. This sort of obsession invariably ends in misery and failure. I've never known a 'food weigher' to diet successfully. The obsession can too easily lead to boredom, dissatisfaction and frustration – as well as an unhealthy concern with food.

23 Don't bother counting calories either. Many diets suggest a special daily calorie allowance of anything from 600 to 1500 calories (2500–6300kj). The trouble is that everyone's calorie needs are different. You won't know how few calories you need to eat to lose weight until you try! Diet books which rely on calorie lists are useless. My method – which relies on you eating when you are hungry and stopping the moment you no longer feel hungry – is guaranteed to help you keep your weight constant for life, while the numerous slimming guidelines and tips contained in this book will help you lose any unwanted weight that you've already accumulated.

24 Don't worry about trying to balance your diet with all the right nutrients. Some slimmers spend hours worrying about protein, minerals and vitamins. If you eat a good, balanced diet your body will look after itself. People managed to avoid getting overweight for thousands of years without even knowing of the existence of protein, minerals or vitamins!

25 If you look at diets in women's magazines you'll often see articles promising that you can lose 7lb (3kg) or even more in a week. These diets are silly, short-term and potentially dangerous. Ignore them. You should aim at losing around 2lb (1kg) a week. If you lose more than that on the 'green' diet that's fine – but as a regular target 2lb (1kg) a week is fine.

26 When eating apples, peaches and pears eat them with the skin on – the skin contains much of the goodness. Wash them well first.

27 Bake potatoes in their skins occasionally – again, the skins are full of goodness.

28 Rice is an excellent – and, in the West, still underused – food. Filling, full of nourishment and low in calories, it makes a great alternative to potatoes.

29 Use sweeteners instead of sugar. These days you can buy them in granulated as well as tablet form. They are often four times as sweet as sugar and can be used on fruit and cereals as well as in drinks. Liquid sweeteners are an excellent alternative to sugar when you are cooking. By substituting them for sugar most people can cut enough calories out of their diet to lose over 14lb (6kg) a year!

30 If you are used to munching lots of sweets – and always having something to chew in your mouth – try sugar-free chewing gum. It isn't a particularly pleasant habit, but it may help you break yourself of the sweet-crunching habit.

31 If you buy fizzy soft drinks, always buy the 'diet' versions that don't contain sugar.

32 Drink plenty of water (bottled water if you don't like or don't trust your tap water). Water contains no calories but will help to keep you full – and will keep your kidneys in tip-top condition.

33 Don't put salt out on the table. Many people sprinkle salt on their food before they have even *tasted* it. Salt can result in fluid retention.

34 Don't spend too much time *looking* at mouth-watering food. There is now evidence to show that you can get fat just by looking! When you see, smell or think of food your body starts to prepare its digestive processes. Saliva is released in your mouth and your stomach produces juices to help digest the coming food. The pancreas is stimulated and insulin is produced. The insulin then starts to convert the glucose in your bloodstream into fat as your body clears the way for the food it thinks is on the way. However, as the amount of sugar circulating in your blood falls so you will begin to feel genuinely hungry. And you'll need to eat. Your body will have been tricked by its own senses.

35 Never make the mistake of rewarding yourself with food – you'll be establishing (or reinforcing) a 'reward habit' which will soon make you fat. Instead, treat yourself to a book, magazine, tape or bunch of flowers. Food is for eating, not rewarding.

36 Persuade friends and relatives not to buy you food (for example, chocolates) as a present.

37 When you go to the shops to buy food take a shopping list with you – and stick to what's on it. Don't be suckered into buying impulse foods at the checkout.

38 Try new foods as often as you can. Look at the fruit and vegetable counter in your local supermarket, for example, and buy small quantities of items you've never tried before. This will add variety and spice to your new diet.

39 Don't buy junk foods. If other members of your family want junk foods, let them buy their own.

40 When out shopping, learn to read the labels on the food you buy. Look for products that are low in fat and other 'dangerous' ingredients.

41 Be sceptical about food advertising. Remember that the big food companies are simply after your money. Learn to read or watch ads critically. Try to analyse them and see how the copywriter is trying to part you from your money.

42 Never nibble while cooking. Many cooks I know kid themselves that they're testing food as they cook. But by the time the meal is ready they will have eaten far more than a 'sample'. This sort of eating has nothing to do with hunger and is dangerous both to your diet and to your health.

43 Avoid frying foods. If you *must* fry, use a non-stick pan so that you don't have to add any extra fat.

44 If you like your salad dressed, either buy or make a low-calorie or no-calorie dressing. You can make your own dressing with wine vinegar and garden herbs – or you can use low-fat yoghurt and herbs.

45 Begin a collection of vegetarian recipes. Changing your eating habits means that many of your old favourites will no longer be usable. But this can be an exciting time – it gives you a chance to learn many new culinary skills.

46 Teach your children good eating habits. Explain to them why some foods are good for them and other foods bad.

47 Never reward children with food for good behaviour or success. You'll be starting a lifetime of problems.

48 Remember that people aren't born with a 'sweet tooth'. We acquire it through experience. Don't fill up your children with a diet of sweets and chocolates.

49 Never make children eat up all the food on their plates if they say they're full. Let them leave food if they can't eat it. If you're worried, talk to your doctor.

50 If someone in your family always leaves food, give them less to start with! It will make you – and them – feel much better.

51 Remember that alcohol is absolutely packed with calories.

52 If you drink tonic water or any other mixer with alcohol, make sure that the barman uses a low-calorie version.

54 If you're eating out, only take enough money with you for the basic foods that you know you'll need. If you only have enough money for a cup of coffee you won't end up succumbing to temptation and buying a cream bun as well.

55 If you buy chips from a fish and chip shop, make sure that they're cooked in low-fat vegetable oil.

56 If you're going out, take your own snacks with you – it'll be cheaper and probably much better for your health. If you suddenly get hungry and you haven't got a snack with you, there is a danger that you'll end up buying a bar of chocolate. The alternative risk is that you'll get back home starving hungry and stuff yourself with whatever comes to hand! Never, *never* let yourself get really hungry – if you do, you'll find it difficult to eat wisely.

57 If it's break-time at work and you don't feel like eating or drinking anything pop outside, go for a quick walk, make a private phone call, write a letter or read a magazine.

58 Find non-fattening ways of dealing with boredom. Get into the habit of doing crosswords, writing letters, tidying the house or gardening when you feel bored. Never use food to distract, entertain or amuse yourself.

59 If you usually keep snacks or sweets in the car, buy nuts and dried fruit rather than chocolates or sugar-rich sweets.

60 Buy individually wrapped biscuits as snacks. They're slightly more expensive, but if you buy an ordinary packet of biscuits there's a real risk that you'll just eat your way through the lot before you know what you're doing.

61 Before you start the 'green' diet have a photograph of yourself taken. Keep it. Looking at it will give you encouragement as you lose weight. (And, who knows, you may be able to use the old 'before' picture to help you win a slimming competition when you've lost weight!)

62 Make up your mind that as soon as you've lost your excess weight you will buy clothes to show off your figure. Be proud of yourself. Better still, start buying clothes *now* that you will only be able to wear when you've lost weight. It's a great incentive!

63 When you lose weight, throw out the clothes that no longer fit you. Keeping them is merely a sign that you don't expect your dieting to be permanent. With the aid of this book your diet is going to work – for ever.

64 If you are receiving treatment for any medical condition tell your doctor before you start this diet – and then visit him regularly while you lose weight. If you need to take medication, there is a good chance that dieting will mean that your treatment can be reduced or even stopped.

65 Many prescribed pills can produce an unwanted weight gain. Drugs such as steroids and the contraceptive pill can all do this. If you're regularly taking any prescribed pill – and you think it could be damaging your attempts at dieting – talk to your doctor. There may be an alternative he can prescribe. If you're taking the contraceptive pill, for example, there will almost certainly be equally effective alternatives that you can try.

66 Some drugs that you can buy over the counter – without a prescription – can also produce a weight gain. Ask your pharmacist or doctor for their advice. And remember that you should never take unprescribed drugs for more than five days without obtaining medical advice.

67 If, having lost excess weight, you're left with stretch marks or folds of unwanted skin, talk to your doctor about the possibility of cosmetic surgery.

68 Don't weigh yourself every day. Once a week is quite enough. Your daily weight will vary enormously for a variety of quite natural reasons.

69 Always weigh yourself at the same time of day – and wearing the same clothes (preferably none at all).

70 Keep a slimming diary and make a record of every pound you've lost. You'll gain constant encouragement from your past successes.

71 Learn how to deal with stress – how to relax properly.

Many people eat when they're under pressure. Make sure you don't.

72 If you want to take up exercise, choose something you'll enjoy. Exercise that you don't enjoy won't work – you'll soon find yourself making excuses not to bother. The four best, safest and most popular forms of exercise among slimmers are walking, swimming, dancing and cycling.

73 Walking is the best exercise you can take – it's good for every part of your body. Try to make sure you walk somewhere every day. Get off the bus a stop early or leave the car at home. Buy yourself some comfortable walking shoes. If you want to change into a smart pair when you arrive at your destination, carry them with you in a bag.

74 If you have difficulty in remembering to eat only when you're hungry, enlist help from your partner and friends. Ask them to remind you that you're eating if they see you eating 'automatically' (for example, nibbling while watching television). Get them to ask you the magic question: 'Are you *really* hungry?'

75 If you have a friend who also wants to lose weight, ring one another up with ideas and support.

76 If you find slimming alone difficult, consider joining a slimming club – there are hundreds in all areas, and slimming magazines and local newspapers will carry details. At a slimming club you'll get encouragement and support from people who understand the problems you're facing.

77 Learn not to be upset if you meet someone who can eat twice as much as you without putting on one extra pound in weight. We are all different. Some people burn up food faster than others. Some people are tall, some are thin. Some are dark-haired, some are blonde. Some naturally burn up food faster than others.

78 Spend a little time analysing your eating habits. Try to work out *why* you have been an over-eater. Think back to when you were a child. Work out how you acquired your bad eating habits. Once you know where your bad habits came from, you'll find it a good deal easier to get rid of them.

79 Sometimes slimmers insist that they have difficulty in listening to their bodies. 'I can't tell when I'm hungry or full!' is a common complaint. It's simply a question of practice.

Don't give up. Whenever you are eating, concentrate hard to decide whether or not you are still hungry. If you find it really difficult, stop eating for a moment while you think. Eventually your appetite control centre will rebuild its strength and you'll automatically know whether or not you're still hungry.

80 Make your right hand into a fist. That is the approximate size of your stomach. Even if you were starving, the amount of food you would need to satisfy your hunger would only fill a container the size of your fist.

81 If you're eating with a group of other people, make sure that you're the last to start. You're probably going to eat less than anyone else, so if you start last you'll be less likely to finish first – and risk drawing attention to the fact that you may not have emptied your plate.

82 Don't keep your diet a secret. Don't force the issue, but if the subject comes up naturally then be prepared to talk about the changes you are making. Never be shy or embarrassed. Explain why you've made the changes you've made. If you try to keep things secret you'll face difficulties and embarrassments when you eat out or invite visitors to your home.

83 Always be positive when talking about your eating habits. If someone says to you: 'Are you trying to diet?' say 'No! I've decided to change my eating habits and lose some weight.' The word 'try' suggests the possibility of failure. You are not going to fail.

84 Make up your mind that you will never again blame anyone else for your weight. *You* control your weight – no one else.

85 Don't listen to people who scoff at your dieting plans. It's *your* body and *your* life. *You* should make the decision about whether or not you diet.

86 Even though you may be proud of your new diet – and your slimming success – don't preach to the unconverted. Talk about your diet, answer people's questions, but don't take a moral stance and never be rude or scornful about people who eat meat. You'll stand a much better chance of winning converts if you give people the facts and allow them to make their own choices. If you annoy or antagonize people you will not only put them off 'eating green' but you will also lose their support and enthusiasm and encouragement. We need all the support, enthusiasm and encouragement we can get.

87 Alcoholics are told to try to live one day at a time when they give up alcohol. Slimmers can often benefit enormously by thinking the same way. Tackle each day as it comes, never think of the past and don't worry too much about the future. If you follow this simple prescription, you'll find slimming success far easier to achieve.

88 If you slip from this dieting programme, don't despair. Everyone has a bad day. Everyone makes a mistake. No one is perfect. Forget it. Instead of worrying about the slip concentrate on making sure that tomorrow your diet goes well.

89 Don't be disappointed if you put a little weight back on again while you're dieting. Don't despair − it often happens. The human body is complicated and your weight is likely to fluctuate regularly. Check to ensure that you aren't making any mistakes, and then just continue with your diet.

90 As your appetite control centre rebuilds its strength you'll probably find yourself occasionally developing a craving for some particular type of food. Don't worry! This is merely a sign that your body is regaining its health. If you suddenly feel that you want to eat an orange or a piece of melon, that's almost certainly what your body *needs*. The food selection mechanisms in the human body are sophisticated and accurate. Most of us are only accustomed to the simpler, crude parts of the mechanism − the parts that tell us that because we've eaten too many salted nuts we need another drink! Oddly, pregnant women are often extremely aware of their body's needs.

91 Once you stop trying to satisfy your emotions with food you'll probably find that these emotions become much more apparent. As you continue with the 'green' diet you'll become much more aware of the ups and downs of life. You may have the odd unhappy day, but you'll also find that you enjoy life far, far more than ever before.

92 As you lose excess weight you'll find that your confidence builds. Use that confidence. Think back to all the things you've wanted to try − but never had the nerve to: learning to sail, modelling, competition dancing, ice skating. . .

93 You'll probably notice that strangers react quite differently to the new slim you. People often treat thin people differently from fat people. Prejudice and expectations colour our actions

more than we like to admit. You'll probably find that friends will treat you differently, too. Be prepared for this.

94 Don't worry if you find you need less sleep when you're dieting. This is common among slimmers – and particularly common among people who have given up red meat. A meat-free diet that is relatively low in fat content usually means that people suffer less from tiredness and exhaustion.

95 Be prepared for the wolf whistles and the compliments. Some successful slimmers are startled – and frightened – when they become exceptionally attractive to members of the opposite sex. They've forgotten how to cope with it. Be prepared!

96 Sort out your fridge and food cupboards every week. Throw out food that is not going to be used.

97 Don't let other people push or manipulate you into eating food you don't want or need.

98 If other members of your family need to lose weight try to persuade them to lose weight with you.

99 Eat most of your meals sitting at the table. You'll find it easier to concentrate on what you are doing — and stop when you're no longer hungry — if you're *not* slumped in front of the TV set with a tray on your lap.

100 If you ever feel doubtful about your ability to succeed, or doubtful about whether or not the 'green' diet is right for *you*, reread the early chapters of this book. Remember that by choosing to 'eat green' you are doing much, much more than simply adopting a new diet; you are making a statement to yourself and, in a quiet but practical way, to the world. You are adopting a new way of life and can take quiet and private satisfaction from the fact that, by choosing to 'eat green', you have helped to make the world a better place to live in.

PART THREE
FOOD AND RECIPES

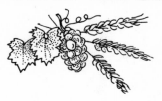

8

The Eat Green Food Fact File

Doctors, dieticians and nutritionists always talk about the importance of having a balanced diet. But how can you tell if you're eating a balanced diet? How do you know whether the foods you're eating contain a good variety of minerals and vitamins? How can you tell whether you're getting enough protein? How do you know whether your diet is as rich in fibre as you know it ought to be? With the aid of this information file you can 'mix and match' your own ingredients and prepare a balanced diet to suit your own tastes.

To help make the whole thing quick and easy to use I've devised a unique star system for all the foods I've listed. Instead of including meaningless and confusing (and often misleading) information about milligrams and percentages I've simply given every food in the file a series of ratings, which will enable you to identify the content and value of a food at a glance. A one-star rating under a particular heading means that the food contains very little or none of that ingredient. A three-star rating means that it's packed with that particular ingredient.

Balancing your diet has never been simpler!

Biscuits

Many bought biscuits contain numerous additives. Plain biscuits – such as digestives and semi-sweet varieties – contain far less sugar than the fancy kinds. Many biscuits contain some minerals, but oatcakes are the only ones to contain minerals in appreciable quantities. Home-made biscuits can be baked with similar amounts of sugar and with more bran than most factory-produced ones.

BISCUITS	Protein	Fat	Fibre	Vitamins & Minerals	Calories
CHOCOLATE	☆	☆☆	☆	☆	☆☆☆
DIGESTIVE	☆	☆	☆☆	☆	☆☆
GINGER	☆	☆	☆	☆	☆☆
OATCAKES	☆	☆	☆☆	☆☆	☆☆
SEMI-SWEET	☆	☆	☆	☆	☆☆
SHORTBREAD	☆	☆☆		☆	☆☆☆

Bread

All bread is good for you – but some types of bread are better than others. Wholemeal bread contains more fibre, but even 'ordinary' white bread contains protein and essential minerals in addition to fibre. Try to choose bread that tastes good – and to eat it as fresh as possible. The better bread tastes, the less likely you are to have to cover it with a thick layer of fatty butter before you can eat it.

BREAD	Protein	Fat	Fibre	Vitamins & Minerals	Calories
BROWN	☆☆	☆	☆☆	☆☆	☆☆
NAAN	☆☆	☆	☆☆	☆☆	☆☆☆
PITTA	☆☆	☆	☆☆	☆☆	☆☆
POPPADUMS	☆	☆	☆☆	☆	☆☆☆
WHITE	☆☆	☆	☆☆	☆☆	☆☆
WHOLEMEAL	☆☆	☆	☆☆☆	☆☆☆	☆☆

Breakfast cereals

Bought breakfast cereals often contain added vitamins and minerals, but they also often include added sugar and salt.

Look at the packet before you buy, and check out the ingredients. The two healthiest breakfast cereals are porridge (made with bran-rich oatmeal) and muesli. Buy your own raw ingredients and prepare your own each week. You can add fresh or dried fruit according to your taste.

BREAKFAST CEREALS	Protein	Fat	Fibre	Vitamins & Minerals	Calories
BRAN	☆	☆	☆☆☆☆	☆	☆
CORNFLAKES	☆	☆	☆☆	☆☆	☆☆☆☆
MUESLI	☆☆	☆☆	☆☆	☆☆	☆☆☆☆
PORRIDGE	☆☆	☆☆	☆☆	☆☆	☆

Cakes, buns and pastries

Most of these items are rich in fat and calories and low in fibre. Some contain minerals – particularly calcium and iron. Surprisingly, a few types of cake (for example cheesecake and sponge cake) contain vitamin A.

CAKE, BUNS & PASTRIES	Protein	Fat	Fibre	Vitamins & Minerals	Calories
CHEESECAKE	☆	☆☆☆	☆	☆☆	☆☆☆
CHOCOLATE CAKE	☆	☆☆☆	☆	☆	☆☆☆
DANISH PASTRIES	☆	☆☆☆	☆	☆	☆☆☆
DOUGHNUTS	☆	☆☆☆	☆	☆	☆☆☆
FRUIT CAKE	☆	☆☆☆	☆	☆	☆☆☆
GINGER CAKE	☆	☆☆☆	☆	☆☆	☆☆☆
MERINGUE	☆	☆☆☆	☆	☆	☆☆☆
MINCE PIES	☆	☆☆☆	☆	☆	☆☆☆
ROCK CAKES	☆	☆☆☆	☆	☆☆	☆☆☆
SPONGE CAKE	☆	☆☆☆	☆	☆☆	☆☆☆

Cheese

Most people who give up meat or cut down their meat consumption eat more cheese. It's easy to create meals and snacks around cheese (pizza, omelettes and cheese sandwiches) and there are many different types available. But do watch out – many cheeses are rich in fat! The table below lists cheeses by type – you can reduce your fat intake by buying low-fat cheeses which are now widely available.

There is one problem with cheese which I haven't yet mentioned. In the preparation of their cheeses many manufacturers use rennet – an extract taken from the stomach linings of cud-chewing animals. Rennet contains an enzyme called rennin which helps to clot the milk and produce the curds from which cheeses are made. There *are* alternatives to animal rennin, and you can buy cheese that hasn't been made with rennet – but not all shops stock such cheeses.

You might like to campaign for shops and restaurants to stock cheeses which haven't been made with rennet. Meanwhile, if you can't find rennet-free cheeses, unless you are a vegan I don't think you should feel bad about eating cheeses which have been made with rennet.

CHEESE	Protein	Fat	Fibre	Vitamins & Minerals	Calories
BRIE	☆☆☆	☆☆	☆	☆☆☆	☆☆
CAMEMBERT	☆☆☆	☆☆	☆	☆☆☆	☆☆
CHEDDAR	☆☆☆	☆☆☆	☆	☆☆☆	☆☆☆
CHESHIRE	☆☆☆	☆☆☆	☆	☆☆☆	☆☆☆
COTTAGE	☆☆☆	☆	☆	☆☆☆	☆
CREAM	☆	☆☆☆	☆	☆☆	☆☆☆
DANISH BLUE	☆☆☆	☆☆☆	☆	☆☆☆	☆☆☆
EDAM	☆☆☆	☆☆	☆	☆☆☆	☆☆
GRUYÈRE	☆☆☆	☆☆☆	☆	☆☆☆	☆☆☆
PARMESAN	☆	☆☆☆	☆	☆☆	☆☆☆
ROQUEFORT	☆☆☆	☆☆☆	☆	☆☆☆	☆☆☆
STILTON	☆☆☆	☆☆☆	☆	☆☆☆	☆☆☆

Dairy products excluding cheese

Milk is good for us — it is high in protein and contains a number of vitamins and minerals, particularly calcium — but most of us drink far too much of it. Each animal species produces milk with which to feed its own young. Cow's milk is different from human milk in that it is richer in protein, fat and minerals. If you think about it, it really isn't all that surprising — a calf which feeds on its mother's milk will reach full size in just two years, whereas a human infant will take sixteen years to reach the equivalent size. Human milk contains more vitamins, a different protein and antibodies which provide protection against different infections.

No adult mammal naturally chooses to drink milk after it has been weaned (indeed, most adults lack one of the enzymes needed to digest it properly). Milk-drinking is in fact a relatively recent Western habit that was largely created as a result of the commercialization of farming. Sadly, there is now a growing amount of evidence to show that milk-drinking is responsible for a wide range of health problems among adults and children. Some experts now claim that three-quarters of all allergies and nearly half of all digestive problems in children are caused by milk.

In recent years farmers and their marketing representatives have worked hard to encourage us all to drink more milk (partly because of huge surpluses — nearly half of the European Community's farm budget goes on storing and getting rid of excess milk). It has, for example, been claimed that the calcium in milk is especially good for women who are going through the menopause and who are particularly liable to suffer from weak and unusually fragile bones. However, the available evidence does *not* support the theory that drinking extra milk will make bones healthier or reduce their risk of breaking. Indeed, the evidence all supports the notion that most of us should make a real effort to drink less milk. Apart from its link to allergy problems such as eczema, asthma and sinus disorders, ordinary milk contains relatively large amounts of fat. Low-fat versions — skimmed and semi-skimmed milks — are now available from most dairies and these seem to be an excellent alternative.

Perhaps most worrying of all is the news that some farmers are now being encouraged to give their cows hormones to increase their milk yield (though why on earth we should be encouraging farmers to produce more milk when many Western countries have a massive surplus of the stuff, I cannot imagine). No one yet knows exactly what effect these hormones will have on you and your family.

Finally, two other points about milk that are worth remembering. First, when some of the fat is taken from milk to produce 'skimmed' or 'semi-skimmed' milk, some of the fat-soluble vitamins A and D go too. The protein and calcium remain. Some dairies do now add extra vitamins to their skimmed milk. Most experts seem to think that babies and children under the age of five who drink milk should be given the ordinary variety rather than skimmed or semi-skimmed – they need the extra calories that ordinary milk contains. Second, if you're allergic to cow's milk then you could try goat's milk or sheep's milk. They are, however, not as widely available as cow's milk and they may contain more fat.

Before leaving the subject of dairy products I must just remind you that butter and margarine are both very high in saturated fats. The widely available low-fat spreads which are becoming increasingly popular contain polyunsaturated fats, which are much safer for you.

BUTTER & MILK	Protein	Fat	Fibre	Vitamins & Minerals	Calories
BUTTER	☆	☆☆☆☆	☆	☆	☆☆☆
LOW-FAT SPREAD	☆	☆☆	☆	☆	☆☆
MARGARINE	☆	☆☆☆☆	☆	☆	☆☆☆
MILK (WHOLE)	☆☆	☆☆☆☆	☆	☆☆☆	☆☆☆
CONDENSED MILK	☆☆	☆☆☆☆	☆	☆☆☆	☆☆☆
SKIMMED MILK	☆☆	☆	☆	☆☆☆	☆
SEMI-SKIMMED MILK	☆☆	☆☆	☆	☆☆☆	☆☆
GOAT'S MILK	☆☆	☆☆☆☆	☆	☆☆	☆☆☆
SHEEP'S MILK	☆☆	☆☆☆☆	☆	☆☆	☆☆☆

Eggs

Since it became widely known that the majority of modern egg-producing hens are contaminated with salmonella, eggs have attracted a considerable amount of adverse publicity. However, the problems aren't quite as bad as they might seem to be. The risk of contracting salmonella poisoning from contaminated eggs is slight – probably one in several million – and only the very young, the very old or the very weak are likely to suffer anything more than a mild digestive upset after contracting salmonella. But most people – particularly people who have given up meat – eat too many of them.

There is surprisingly little goodness in eggs, which contain small amounts of protein and tiny quantities of iron but are rich in cholesterol. Very few foods contain *more* cholesterol than eggs. My advice is not to eat more than two or three eggs a week. Buy free-range eggs rather than those laid by hens kept in battery cages (and if possible ask for your eggs to be packed in reusable and eventually biodegradable cardboard containers rather than plastic non-degradable containers).

	Protein	Fat	Fibre	Vitamins & Minerals	Calories
EGGS	☆	☆☆☆	☆	☆	☆☆☆

Fish

An excellent substitute for meat, fish are rich in vitamins and polyunsaturates but contain few saturated fats. All fish contain phosphorous, and most seafish contain iodine. Small fish which are eaten whole (such as whitebait and sardines) are good sources of calcium. Oily fish such as mackerel, herrings, tuna and salmon contain essential fatty acids and fat-soluble vitamins such as A and D. All fish contain the B vitamins. White fish such as cod, haddock, plaice and sole are very low in calories (though frying can double the number of calories eaten). Many fish are rich in iron: sardines contain as much iron as many meats, and fried sprats contain more than steak.

Shellfish such as oysters, cockles, mussels, whelks, prawns and crab all contain about the same amount of protein and fat as white fish – and have a roughly similar vitamin content. Their calorie content is similar. Oysters are a rich source of zinc.

Fish products such as fish fingers and fish cakes are high in saturated fat. They may also contain a wide number of ingredients in addition to fish.

FISH	Protein	Fat	Fibre	Vitamins & Minerals	Calories
COD	☆☆☆	☆	☆	☆☆	☆☆
CRAB	☆☆☆	☆	☆	☆☆☆	☆☆
HERRINGS	☆☆☆	☆☆	☆	☆☆☆	☆☆☆
KIPPERS	☆☆☆	☆☆	☆	☆☆☆	☆☆☆
MACKEREL	☆☆☆	☆☆	☆	☆☆☆	☆☆☆
PILCHARDS	☆☆☆	☆☆	☆	☆☆☆	☆☆
PLAICE	☆☆☆	☆	☆	☆☆☆	☆☆
PRAWNS	☆☆☆	☆	☆	☆☆☆	☆☆
SALMON	☆☆☆	☆☆	☆	☆☆☆	☆☆☆
TROUT	☆☆☆	☆☆	☆	☆☆	☆☆
TUNA	☆☆☆	☆☆	☆	☆☆☆	☆☆☆
FISH CAKES	☆☆	☆☆	☆	☆☆	☆☆☆
FISH FINGERS	☆☆	☆☆	☆	☆☆	☆☆☆

The high price of salmon and trout means that fish farming is now big business. Inevitably, perhaps, fish farmers use hormones to make their fish grow faster, antibiotics to help control infection and other chemicals to control infestation. In addition some fish farmers treat their competitors rather ruthlessly – every year thousands of seals, cormorants and herons which might be a threat are killed. Additional damage

to the environment — and undoubted cruelty to the fish
themselves — means that many thoughtful fish-eaters now
avoid eating fish that have been reared on special 'farms'.

Food poisoning from eating 'bad' fish is rare. Fish that has
gone 'off' smells so bad that few people would dream of eating
it.

Fruit

No diet can be complete without a good, regular supply of
fruit. Fresh is best. If you buy tinned fruit, try to buy
unsweetened varieties that contain no additives. Dried fruits
make excellent snacks. Many canned and dried fruits still
contain minerals and vitamins, but the best supplies of these
essentials are usually to be found in fresh products.

FRUIT	Protein	Fat	Fibre	Vitamins & Minerals	Calories
APPLES	☆	☆	☆☆	☆☆	☆
APRICOTS	☆	☆	☆☆	☆☆	☆
AVOCADOS	☆	☆☆☆☆	☆☆	☆☆	☆☆☆
BANANAS	☆	☆	☆☆	☆☆☆☆	☆
BLACKBERRIES	☆	☆	☆☆☆☆	☆☆☆☆	☆
CHERRIES	☆	☆	☆☆	☆☆	☆
FIGS	☆	☆	☆☆	☆☆	☆
GRAPEFRUIT	☆	☆	☆	☆☆☆☆	☆
GRAPES	☆	☆	☆	☆☆	☆☆
LEMONS	☆	☆	☆	☆☆☆☆	☆
MANGOES	☆	☆	☆☆	☆☆	☆☆
MELONS	☆	☆	☆	☆☆☆☆	☆
ORANGES	☆	☆	☆	☆☆☆☆	☆
PEACHES	☆	☆	☆	☆☆	☆
PEARS	☆	☆	☆	☆☆	☆
PINEAPPLES	☆	☆	☆	☆☆☆☆	☆
PLUMS	☆	☆	☆	☆☆	☆
RAISINS (DRIED)	☆	☆	☆	☆☆	☆☆
STRAWBERRIES	☆	☆	☆	☆☆	☆

Nuts and seeds

Apart from peanuts (raw or salted), most non-vegetarians only ever think of eating nuts at parties. That's a pity. There are many different kinds of nuts and seeds available and most are terrific when served whole in salads, used to enliven a breakfast cereal, as snacks or when mashed up to make spreads. If your usual grocery store doesn't stock many nuts, try visiting a health food store.

Incidentally I'm well aware that, strictly speaking, peanuts are pulses and should be listed along with peas and beans – but since most of us think of them as nuts I've included them here.

NUTS	Protein	Fat	Fibre	Vitamins & Minerals	Calories
ALMONDS	☆☆	☆☆☆☆	☆	☆	☆☆☆
BRAZIL NUTS	☆	☆☆☆☆	☆	☆☆	☆☆☆
CASHEWS	☆☆	☆☆☆☆	☆	☆☆	☆☆☆
CHESTNUTS	☆	☆	☆	☆	☆☆
COCONUT	☆	☆☆☆☆	☆	☆	☆☆☆
HAZELNUTS (FILBERTS)	☆	☆☆☆☆	☆	☆	☆☆☆
PEANUTS	☆☆	☆☆☆☆	☆	☆☆	☆☆☆
PECAN NUTS	☆	☆☆☆☆	☆	☆	☆☆☆
WALNUTS	☆	☆☆☆	☆	☆	☆☆☆
SESAME SEEDS	☆☆	☆☆☆☆	☆	☆☆	☆☆☆
SUNFLOWER SEEDS	☆☆	☆☆☆	☆	☆☆	☆☆☆

Pasta

When people think of pasta they usually think of ordinary white spaghetti – but there's far more to pasta than that! Look around in your local store and you'll see that there are dozens of different varieties of pasta – suitable for a huge variety of different recipes (none of which need involve meats). Remember, too, that wholemeal pasta contains more fibre, more protein, more vitamins and more minerals than ordinary white pasta.

PASTA	Protein	Fat	Fibre	Vitamins & Minerals	Calories
SPAGHETTI (WHITE)	☆	☆	☆	☆	☆
SPAGHETTI (WHOLEMEAL)	☆☆	☆	☆☆	☆☆	☆

Poultry

Sometimes known as 'white' meat, poultry is a halfway point between meat-eating and vegetarianism. If you want to give up red meat but aren't happy about giving up meat altogether, eating poultry is a sensible compromise. Most types contain considerably less fat than most types of red meat, and although chicken is more likely to be infected with salmonella (and therefore needs to be prepared with some care) the health risks associated with white meat are considerably less than those associated with red meat.

Remember, by the way, that most of the fat associated with poultry is found in and just underneath the skin. If you avoid the skin and eat just the meat then you reduce your fat – and calorie – consumption considerably.

POULTRY	Protein	Fat	Fibre	Vitamins & Minerals	Calories
CHICKEN	☆☆☆	☆☆	☆	☆☆	☆☆
DUCK	☆☆☆	☆☆☆	☆	☆☆	☆☆☆
TURKEY	☆☆☆	☆☆	☆	☆☆	☆☆

Puddings and sweets

These are often the downfall of dieters – largely because most would-be slimmers have, over the years, acquired at least one sweet tooth! There may well, however, be a few surprises on this list. . .

PUDDINGS & SWEETS	Protein	Fat	Fibre	Vitamins & Minerals	Calories
BREAD PUDDING	☆☆	☆☆	☆☆	☆☆☆	☆☆☆
CHOCOLATE PUDDING	☆	☆☆☆☆	☆	☆	☆☆☆
FRUIT PIE	☆	☆☆	☆	☆☆	☆☆☆
FRUIT SALAD (FRESH)	☆	☆	☆	☆☆	☆
ICE CREAM	☆	☆☆☆☆	☆	☆☆	☆☆☆
JELLY	☆	☆	☆	☆	☆
PANCAKES	☆☆	☆☆	☆	☆☆	☆☆☆
RICE PUDDING	☆	☆	☆	☆☆	☆☆
TRIFLE	☆	☆☆☆☆	☆	☆☆	☆☆☆
YOGHURT (NATURAL)	☆☆	☆	☆	☆☆☆	☆
YOGHURT (FLAVOURED)	☆☆	☆	☆	☆☆☆	☆☆

Pulses (legumes)

One of the most nutritious meals in the world is also one of the simplest – baked beans on wholemeal toast. Beans are probably the best-known member of the pulse family, but others include peas, lentils, soya and tofu. Pulses are an essential part of the 'green' diet.

PULSES (LEGUMES)	Protein	Fat	Fibre	Vitamins & Minerals	Calories
BAKED BEANS	☆☆	☆	☆☆	☆☆☆	☆
BROAD BEANS	☆☆	☆	☆☆	☆☆☆	☆
BUTTER BEANS	☆☆	☆	☆☆	☆☆☆	☆
FRENCH BEANS	☆	☆	☆☆	☆☆☆	☆
RUNNER BEANS	☆	☆	☆☆	☆☆☆	☆
LENTILS	☆☆	☆	☆☆	☆☆☆	☆
SOYA BEANS	☆☆☆	☆☆	☆☆	☆☆☆	☆

Grains (oats, rice and wheat)

Oats are one of the most useful foods available for the vegetarian and the slimmer. If you're a vegetarian *and* a slimmer, then they should definitely always be on your shopping list. Oat bran contains protein, carbohydrate and vitamin B – as well as more soluble fibre than any other food. Oatmeal contains the same basic ingredients – but rather less fibre. Oats have several vital functions:

a they slow down the passage of food so that you don't feel so hungry so often or so quickly after eating, and thus help slimmers lose weight;

b the digestion of fibre-rich foods uses up energy, oats burn up calories;

c oats – particularly oat bran – will help lower your blood cholesterol level.

For breakfast you can eat oats as porridge. At other times of the day you can eat your oats in bread, biscuits or buns. There is a useful recipe on page 184, but the packets in which oat bran and oatmeal are packed often offer good baking suggestions.

Remember, if you have a high blood cholesterol level or have eaten large amounts of fat in the past, eating oat bran may help your blood clear out some of the superfluous fat.

The *best-known* grain is, of course, rice – a food which is still widely under-used in Western countries although it has for a long time been a basic part of most Eastern diets. Brown rice is much more useful nutritionally than white rice. Other grains include barley, buckwheat, cornmeal, rye and wheat.

GRAINS (OATS, RICE & WHEAT)	Protein	Fat	Fibre	Vitamins & Minerals	Calories
OAT BRAN	☆☆	☆	☆☆☆☆	☆☆☆☆	☆☆
OATMEAL	☆☆	☆	☆☆	☆☆☆☆	☆☆
POPCORN	☆	☆	☆☆	☆	☆☆☆☆
RICE (BROWN)	☆	☆	☆☆	☆☆☆☆	☆☆
RICE (WHITE)	☆	☆	☆	☆☆	☆☆
WHEAT (WHITE)	☆	☆	☆☆	☆☆	☆☆
WHEAT (WHOLE)	☆☆	☆	☆☆☆	☆☆☆☆	☆☆

Vegetables and salads

Almost all vegetables are better for you if eaten raw. All are better for you if they are not cooked to a pulp. Try to eat potatoes baked in their jackets occasionally.

VEGETABLES & SALADS	Protein	Fat	Fibre	Vitamins & Minerals	Calories
ARTICHOKES JERUSALEM OR GLOBE	☆☆	☆	☆☆	☆☆	☆
ASPARAGUS	☆☆	☆	☆☆	☆☆	☆
BAMBOO SHOOTS	☆☆	☆	☆☆	☆☆	☆
BEANSPROUTS	☆	☆	☆	☆	☆
BEETROOT	☆	☆	☆	☆☆	☆
BROCCOLI	☆☆	☆	☆☆	☆☆☆	☆
BRUSSEL SPROUTS	☆☆	☆	☆☆	☆☆☆	☆
CABBAGE	☆☆	☆	☆☆	☆☆☆	☆
CARROTS	☆	☆	☆☆☆	☆☆	☆
CAULIFLOWER	☆☆	☆	☆☆	☆☆☆	☆
CELERY	☆	☆	☆	☆☆	☆
CORN ON THE COB	☆	☆	☆	☆☆	☆☆
CUCUMBER	☆	☆	☆	☆	☆
KALE	☆☆	☆☆	☆☆	☆☆☆	☆
LEEKS	☆	☆	☆	☆☆☆	☆
LETTUCE	☆	☆	☆	☆	☆
MUSHROOMS	☆☆	☆	☆	☆	☆
OLIVES	☆	☆☆☆	☆	☆	☆☆
ONIONS	☆	☆	☆	☆☆	☆
PARSLEY	☆	☆	☆	☆☆	☆
PARSNIPS	☆	☆	☆☆	☆☆	☆
POTATOES	☆	☆	☆☆	☆☆	☆☆
RADISHES	☆	☆	☆	☆	☆
SPINACH	☆☆	☆	☆☆	☆☆☆	☆
TOMATOES	☆	☆	☆	☆	☆
TURNIPS	☆	☆	☆☆	☆☆	☆
WATERCRESS	☆☆	☆	☆	☆☆	☆

9

The Eat Green Recipes

There are hundreds of books which contain recipes suitable for vegetarians of all shades of green. Planning a diet that doesn't include red meat or meat products is really easy. On the following pages are some simple recipes I've prepared to help show you just how exciting and varied the *Eat Green* diet can be. I suggest that you mix'n'match these recipes with others from your own cookery books.

To follow the *Eat Green* diet you don't have to count your calories, weight your food or follow a strict eating pattern. Slimmers will find they have more freedom – and more fun – than ever before!

QUESTION: *I'm very busy – isn't it true that vegetarian food takes longer to prepare than meat dishes?*

ANSWER: *No – it's not true! To begin with you may take longer to prepare vegetarian dishes because they are new to you. But most vegetarian food is quick to prepare and can be easily done in advance.*

QUESTION: *I'd like to stop eating meat but my husband wouldn't dream of it. What can I do?*

ANSWER: *You don't have to eat the same food as your husband any more than you have to vote the same way. Some women I know are vegetarian but still cook meat for their husbands and children. Others cook the rest of the food but insist that the meat-eaters cook the meat.*

Light Green Recipes

These recipes include poultry or fish

Chicken sausages

Makes about 8 sausages

1lb/500g minced chicken meat
1 tablespoon oat bran
pinch of any of the following dried herbs: basil, oregano, sage,
thyme (or whatever else you have handy)

Preheat the oven to 200°C (400°F/gas mark 6) and grease a
baking tray. Mix the meat with the bran and herbs and fashion
the mixture into small 'sausage' shapes on the baking tray.
Cook for 30 minutes.

Chicken and leek casserole

Serves 2

½ pint/300ml cold milk
1 tablespoon cornflour
1 tablespoon grated Parmesan cheese
1 teaspoon French mustard
2 portions cooked chicken (without skin)
2 large leeks, washed and cleaned
1 thick slice stale wholemeal bread

Preheat the oven to 180°C (350°F/gas mark 4) and grease an
ovenproof casserole. Put the milk into a jug and add the
cornflour, stirring until it is a smooth, creamy consistency.
Pour into a heavy saucepan and heat gently, then add the
cheese and mustard – stirring well. Cut the chicken into small
pieces. Cut the leeks into bite-sized chunks and lay them on
the bottom of the casserole. Put the chicken pieces on top of
the leeks and then pour the hot cheese sauce on top. Crumb
the bread and sprinkle the breadcrumbs on top of the
casserole. Cook, uncovered, for 30 minutes.

Green chicken

Serves 2

12oz/350g crisply cooked broccoli
½ pint/300ml vegetable stock
2 large mushrooms, sliced
1 tablespoon arrowroot, dissolved in 1 tablespoon cold water
6 tablespoons skimmed milk
1 teaspoonful finely chopped thyme leaves
1 sage leaf, finely chopped
1½oz/40g low-fat cheese, grated
½ teaspoon soya sauce
4oz/125g cooked chicken breast, thinly sliced

Preheat the oven to 220°C (425°F/gas mark 7). Grease a baking tray and arrange the broccoli on the bottom. Heat the stock, add the mushrooms and simmer for 5 minutes. Add the arrowroot slowly, stirring briskly all the time, then add the milk, herbs, cheese and soya sauce. Simmer for a few minutes. Pour half the sauce over the broccoli and arrange the sliced chicken on top then cover with the remaining sauce. Bake uncovered for 15 minutes.

Victorian kedgeree

Serves 2

3 tablespoons cooked brown rice
2oz/60g cooked, flaked cod
1 tomato, sliced and chopped into small pieces
vegetable oil for frying
1 hard-boiled egg, chopped

Mix together the rice, cod and tomato. Heat a small quantity of vegetable oil in a saucepan. Add the mixture and heat thoroughly, stirring. Serve hot, garnished with chopped hard-boiled egg.

Spaghetti Napoletana

Serves 2

3oz/90g wholemeal spaghetti
1 tablespoon vegetable oil
2oz/60g mushrooms, chopped
½ green pepper, chopped
1 small carrot, chopped
1 small clove garlic, crushed
1 small onion, chopped
4oz/250g tinned tomatoes
1 tablespoon tomato puree
herbs and seasoning to taste
1 tablespoon Parmesan cheese

Cook the spaghetti in boiling water. Fry the vegetables in oil for 5 minutes. Add the tomatoes, the tomato puree and herbs and seasoning to taste. Cook for a few more minutes. Drain the spaghetti and serve with the thick vegetable sauce poured over it, topped with the Parmesan cheese.

Wild chicken

Serves 2

1 tablespoon vegetable oil
2 chicken breasts, skinned, washed and dried
1 medium onion, chopped
1 small cooking apple, chopped
1 clove garlic, crushed
1 tablespoon curry powder
½ teaspoon ground cinnamon
½ teaspoon ground ginger
1 tablespoon mango chutney
¼ pint/150ml skimmed milk

Heat the oil in a saucepan and sauté the chicken until brown. Remove chicken from pan and keep it in a warm place. Add the onion, apple and garlic to the pan and fry until golden. Stir in the curry powder, cinnamon, ginger, chutney and milk. Bring to the boil, return the chicken to the pan and simmer, covered, for 45 minutes or until the chicken is tender.

Turkey barbecue burger

Makes 4 burgers

1lb/500g minced turkey breast
4 tablespoons oat bran
4 tablespoons chopped onion
2 tablespoons chopped mixed peppers

Mix all the ingredients together, make into four burger shapes and grill. Serve with salad garnish and wholemeal buns.

Fish on a stick

Serves 2

4oz/125g cod
½ small red *or* green pepper
1 small onion
2oz/60g button mushrooms
4 tablespoons dry white wine
1½ tablespoons sunflower oil
½ small lemon, cut into quarters

Cut the cod into cubes, the pepper into squares and the onion into quarters. Push alternate pieces of fish, mushroom, pepper and onion on to two skewers. Mix the wine and sunflower oil, pour the mixture over the kebabs and leave for an hour, turning occasionally. Preheat the grill to high. Put the kebabs on to the grill pan and cook for 5–6 minutes, turning regularly. Put a lemon quarter on the end of each skewer.

Fishcakes

Makes about 6 fishcakes

8oz/250g cooked cod (make sure all bones are removed)
8oz/250g cold, boiled potato
1oz/30g polyunsaturated low-fat spread
1 tablespoon chopped parsley

Mash the fish and the potatoes. Mix together with the low-fat spread and parsley. Make into burger shapes and fry in vegetable oil for 3 – 4 minutes.

Cod casserole

Serves 2

½ green pepper
1 leek
2 tomatoes
1 tablespoon vegetable oil
¼ pint/150ml tomato juice
8oz/250g cod with bones removed
1 tablespoon fresh lemon juice
1 tablespoon chopped parsley

Preheat the oven to 180°C (350°F/gas mark 4) and grease a casserole dish. Chop the pepper and leek into small pieces and cut the tomatoes into quarters. Heat the oil in a pan and stir-fry the leek and peppers for 8 minutes, adding the tomato juice after 4 minutes. Remove the pan from the heat and add the quartered tomatoes. Put the vegetables into the bottom of the casserole dish. Cut the fish into small pieces and add them to the dish. Pour the lemon juice over the fish and sprinkle the parsley on top. Cook covered for 15–20 minutes.

Fisherman's pie

Serves 2

3 medium potatoes
¼ pint/150ml skimmed milk *plus* a little extra for mashing
potatoes
1 teaspoon polyunsaturated low-fat spread
1 hard-boiled egg
8oz/250g fresh haddock *or* cod
1 tablespoon cornflour
1 teaspoon fresh chopped parsley
seasoning to taste

Boil the potatoes and mash them with a little skimmed milk
and the low-fat spread. Chop up the hard-boiled egg. Preheat
the oven to 190°C (375°F/gas mark 5) and grease a pie dish. In
a saucepan poach the fish in water for 15 minutes. Remove
and discard the skin and bones, and flake the flesh. Mix the
cornflour with a little cold milk to make a smooth paste. Pour
the remaining milk into a heavy saucepan over a low heat, add
the cornflour and stir well until thickened. Add the egg and
parsley, and spices and pepper according to taste. Mix the
sauce with the fish and put into the pie dish. Arrange the
mashed potatoes on top. Bake for 25 minutes until brown.

Spanish prawns

Serves 2

½ large onion, chopped
1 clove garlic, crushed
2 tablespoons vegetable oil
½ red *or* green pepper
4oz/125g brown rice
4 tablespoons white wine
4 tablespoons vegetable stock
1½ tablespoons tomato puree
½ tablespoon chopped fresh parsley
½ teaspoon dried tarragon
3oz/90g mushrooms
8oz/250g shelled prawns

Preheat the oven to 200°C(400°F/gas mark 6) and grease an ovenproof casserole. Sauté the onion and garlic in 1 tablespoon of the oil, then cut the pepper into thin strips and add it to the pan. Mix in the rice, then add the wine and simmer for 2 minutes. Add all the remaining ingredients except the mushrooms and prawns and bring to the boil. Pour the mixture into the casserole, cover and bake for 50 minutes. Slice the mushrooms. Heat the remaining tablespoon of oil and sauté the mushrooms for 2 minutes, then remove them from the pan and cook the prawns for 2 – 3 minutes. Remove the rice from the oven, mix in the prawns and mushrooms, and return the casserole to the oven for another 5 minutes.

Medium green recipes

These recipes include eggs and dairy products

Venetian Eggs

Serves 2

8oz/250g spinach
1 tablespoon grated Parmesan cheese
2 eggs

Preheat the oven to 180° (350°F/gas mark 4) and grease a small baking dish. Chop the spinach finely and cook in a little water. Spread the spinach over the bottom of the baking dish and sprinkle the cheese on top. Use the back of a spoon to hollow out two dips in the surface of the spinach. Break an egg into each hollow, and bake for 8–10 minutes.

QUESTION: *If I become a vegetarian what do I do when guests are coming to dinner? Or when I've been invited out to a meal?*

ANSWER: *You have to tell them that you're a vegetarian. If you have guests coming to eat with you, explain that they won't be getting any meat or fish. If you're going to eat with other people, then give them plenty of warning. Don't ring up the night before, don't turn up and announce that you're vegetarian when you smell the roast, and don't try to pick your way through a meal without telling anyone. These days there are so many vegetarians that it's easy – though you may have to put up with a few funny looks and snide comments from people who don't understand why you've given up meat. It's up to you whether you want to explain why you don't eat meat. If you become a vegetarian you'll never be short of a topic for conversation – but you will run the risk of becoming a prize bore!*

Parisian salad

Serves 2

I orange, peeled and segmented
1 carrot, grated
½oz/15g almonds, chopped
2oz/60g cottage cheese
2oz/60g celery, chopped
1 stick French bread

Break the orange segments in half, then mix first five ingredients together. Eat with the French bread stick.

Traveller's sandwich

Serves 1–2

1 hard-boiled egg, finely chopped
2oz/60g cottage cheese
4 tablespoons chopped cress
French mustard to taste
½ small wholemeal loaf

Mix the first four ingredients together and use as a sandwich filling.

Savoury Dutch cakes

Serves 2

8oz/250g potatoes, cooked in their skins
nutmeg to taste
ground black pepper to taste
1 tablespoon skimmed milk
1 medium onion, finely chopped
4oz/125g cooked green vegetables

If you intend to use the oven, preheat to 180°C (350°F/gas mark 4) and grease a baking tray. Peel the potatoes then mash with the nutmeg and black pepper. Add the skimmed milk. Fry the onion without oil in a non-stick pan until tender. Mix together the potatoes, green vegetables and onion and form them into four round cakes. Bake for 10 minutes or grill under a moderate heat for 15 minutes.

Golden vegetable parcels

Serves 2

¼ pint/150ml skimmed milk
½ tablespoon cornflour
½ tablespoon chopped parsley
black pepper to taste
selection of leftover cooked vegetables
4oz/125g shortcrust puff pastry

Preheat the oven to 220°C (425°F/gas mark 7) and grease a baking tray. Mix cornflour with a little cold milk to make a smooth paste. Pour remaining milk into a saucepan add cornflour and heat slowly, and stir. Keep the milk on the heat until it has thickened, then add the parsley and season with black pepper. Add the cooked vegetables. Roll out the pastry on a floured surface and cut it into four squares. Put the vegetables into the centres of two of the pastry squares. Brush the edges of the squares with water, and then put the remaining squares on top to make 'parcels'. Pinch the edges together well to seal them. Transfer the parcels to the baking tray and bake for 25 minutes.

L.A. pizza

Serves 2

½ large onion
small tin tomatoes
2 pieces pitta bread
2oz/60g low-fat cheese, grated
dried Italian seasoning – basil, oregano, marjoram, thyme – to
taste
ground black pepper to taste

Soften the onion in a little water over a low heat, but do not brown. Chop up the tomatoes and spread evenly over each piece of pitta bread. Add a layer of onion over the tomato. Sprinkle the cheese over, and top with the herbs and black pepper. Grill until the cheese is golden.

French broccoli

Serves 2

1 tablespoon vegetable oil
2 spring onions, chopped
1 clove garlic, crushed
½ teaspoon oregano
½ teaspoon tarragon
1 tablespoon freshly chopped parsley
pinch cayenne pepper
ground black pepper to taste
12oz/350g cooked broccoli
2oz/60g breadcrumbs
2oz/60g low-fat cheese, grated

Heat the oil and sauté the onions and garlic. Add the herbs and seasonings and then the broccoli. Put the mixture into a fireproof casserole. Mix the breadcrumbs and cheese and place them on top. Grill until the top appears well browned.

Hot devilled eggs

Serves 2

2 hard-boiled eggs
1 tablespoon plain yoghurt
2oz/60g cottage cheese
ground black pepper to taste
pinch of dry mustard powder
paprika to taste

Shell the eggs and cut in half lengthways. Carefully remove
the yolks with sharp knife and put to one side for use in
another dish, or as a sandwich filling. Mix together the
yoghurt and cottage cheese, add the pepper and mustard and
mix until smooth. Spoon the mixture into egg white hollows
and sprinkle lightly with paprika.

Milanese peppers

Serves 2

1 large red *or* green pepper
1 tablespoon vegetable oil
1 large onion, chopped
1 clove garlic, crushed
2 tablespoons red wine
1 tablespoon tomato puree
1 tablespoon mixed chopped rosemary, oregano, parsley
and mint
4 tablespoons vegetable stock
4oz/125g pasta shapes, uncooked
1½oz/40g breadcrumbs
1 egg white
2oz/60g low-fat cheese, grated

Preheat the oven to 180°C (350°F/gas mark 4) and grease a
baking dish. Boil the pepper in water for 1 minute. Then cool it

under running water, halve and remove the seeds. Heat the oil and sauté the onion and garlic. Add the wine, tomato puree, herbs and stock. Simmer for 10 minutes. Place the pasta shapes in a large bowl. Add the breadcrumbs and egg white, mix well, then add the cooked onion and herbs. Spoon the mixture into the pepper halves and place on a baking dish. Put the entire baking dish into a shallow tray containing a little water. Cover, and bake for 20 minutes. Then remove the lid and add the cheese. Bake for another 15 minutes until the peppers are cooked and the cheese is golden.

Oat bran muffins

Makes about 12 American-style muffins
(small cakes, not muffins for toasting)

12oz/350g oat bran
1½oz/40g mixed dried fruit
(raisins, sultanas, currants, chopped dates, etc)
1 tablespoon baking powder
1½oz/40g chopped, mixed nuts
2oz/60g sugar *or* equivalent artificial sweetener
8 fl oz/250ml skimmed milk
2 tablespoons vegetable oil
2 egg whites

Preheat the oven to 220°C (425°F/gas mark 7) and grease a 12-hole deep patty tin. Mix the oat bran, dried fruit, baking powder and nuts, then add the sugar. Mix the milk, oil and egg whites together and add to the oat bran mixture. Mix thoroughly and spoon the mixture evenly into the patty tins. Bake for 15 – 20 minutes or until muffins are firm to press.

Nut biscuits

Makes about 10 biscuits

rice paper
2 egg whites
4oz/125g ground mixed nuts
3oz/90g sugar
2 tablespoons ground brown rice
grated rind of an orange

Preheat the oven to 180°C (350°F/gas mark 4). Grease a baking tray and line it with rice paper. Whisk the egg whites until stiff. Add the nuts and sugar, then stir in the rice and orange rind. Place dollops of the mixture (allow them space to expand during baking) on the rice paper, and cook for 20 – 25 minutes. Serve biscuits each with their square of rice paper.

Natural muesli mix

Serves 2

2 tablespoons oat bran
½ tablespoon sesame seeds
½ tablespoon sunflower seeds
1 apple, sliced
1 banana, sliced
2 tablespoons mixed raisins, sultanas and currants

Mix all the ingredients together well and serve with skimmed milk or plain yoghurt.

Fruity yoghurt

Serves 2

½ pint/300ml plain yoghurt
1 apple, diced
1 orange, peeled and segmented
1 small bunch seedless grapes
¼ small melon, diced
1 banana, sliced
4 tablespoons oat bran

Mix all the ingredients together in a large bowl. Serve chilled.

Dark green recipes

These recipes include only 'pure' vegetarian ingredients

Vegetable hotpot

Serves 2

1 tablespoon vegetable oil
1 medium onion
1 small turnip, sliced
1 small parsnip, sliced
1 large carrot, sliced
1 medium potato, sliced
4 sprouts, sliced
1 pint/600ml water
1 tablespoon soya sauce
1 tablespoon chopped fresh parsley

In a heavy saucepan fry the onion in the oil. Add the rest of the vegetables and half the water. Bring to the boil, then simmer covered for 20 minutes. Add the remaining water and the soya sauce. Just before serving add the parsley.

Devon pasties

Makes 6 pasties

3oz/90g solid vegetable fat (chilled)
4oz/125g wholewheat flour
½ cup cold water
8oz/250g spinach
½ tablespoon olive oil
½ onion, peeled and chopped
½ clove garlic, crushed
1oz/30g breadcrumbs
3oz/90g ground mixed nuts
1 tablespoon chopped parsley

Grate the fat into the flour in a mixing bowl, then add the water and work into a dough. Cover the dough and put in the fridge for 30 minutes. Preheat the oven to 220°C (425°F/gas mark 7) and grease a baking tray. Chop the spinach finely and cook in minimum water for 5 minutes. Cool and puree. Heat the olive oil and fry the onion and garlic. Remove from the heat and then add the breadcrumbs, nuts, parsley and spinach. Roll out the pastry on a floured surface, and cut it into six circles. Share out the filling among the circles and then seal up the pastry, making small holes in each side to allow air to escape during cooking. Bake for 20 minutes.

Royal salad

Serves 2

1 cos lettuce
2 carrots
2 tomatoes
4 radishes
2oz/60g mushrooms
4 spring onions
½ small green pepper
1 apple
2 tablespoons vegetable oil
1 tablespoon cider vinegar
2oz/60g walnut pieces
1oz/30g roasted peanuts
1oz/30g raisins

Shred the lettuce. Grate and chop the vegetables and slice the apple. Combine the oil and vinegar to make a dressing and mix well with the salad. Finally, add the nuts and raisins.

Welsh mushrooms

Serves 2

½ onion, finely chopped
1 clove garlic, finely chopped
1 tablespoon vegetable oil
8oz/250g mushrooms, chopped
dash of soya sauce
2 slices wholemeal toast

Sauté the onion and garlic in the oil. Add the mushrooms to the pan and cook gently. Stir in the soya sauce. Serve on hot toast.

Spaghetti Verona

Serves 2

oil for frying
1 onion, chopped
1 stick celery, chopped
2 tablespoons red wine
12oz/390g tin tomatoes
1 tablespoon tomato puree
1 teaspoon dried mixed Italian herbs
¼ pint/150ml vegetable stock
6oz/175g wholewheat spaghetti

Heat the oil in a frying pan and add the onion and celery. Add
the wine and bring to the boil. Simmer for a few minutes and
add the tomatoes, tomato puree and seasoning. Pour in the
stock and simmer for 30 minutes. Cook the spaghetti according
to the instructions on the packet, and serve immediately with
the hot sauce poured over it.

Portuguese hotpot

Serves 2

1 large potato
1 turnip
1 carrot
1 parsnip
1 onion
4oz/125g French beans
1 clove garlic
¼ pint/150ml vegetable stock
1 teaspoon lemon juice
4 tomatoes, quartered

Coarsely chop all the vegetables (except the tomatoes) and boil
them together. Drain, and add the vegetable stock and lemon

juice. Mix well and continue to cook over a low heat. When the vegetables are just about ready, add the chopped tomatoes. Cook until vegetables ready and tomatoes warmed through.

Russian chilli

Serves 2

½ large onion, chopped
1 tablespoon vegetable oil
4oz/125g burghul (or bulgur) wheat
1 large tin tomatoes
1 tablespoon tomato puree
1 teaspoon chilli powder
ground black pepper to taste
½ large tin red kidney beans *or* 1 small tin

Sauté the onion in the oil. Add the remaining ingredients except the kidney beans and simmer for 20 minutes or until the wheat is cooked but still firm. Add the kidney beans and heat through well.

Pilot's pie

Serves 2

1 tablespoon vegetable oil
3oz/90g onion, chopped
3oz/90g carrot, grated
½ teaspoon dried thyme
½ tablespoon wholemeal flour
½ teaspoon yeast extract
4oz/125g shortcrust pastry
(made with polyunsaturated spread)

Preheat the oven to 190°C (375°F/gas mark 5) and grease a baking dish. Heat the oil and sauté the onion, then add the carrot and thyme and cook gently for 10 minutes. Stir in the flour and yeast extract. Leave to cool. Roll out the pastry and line the dish with half the pastry and pile the filling into the centre. Put the remaining pastry on top and seal the edges. Make two ar three small slits in the top of the pie and bake for 30 minutes.

Greek tomatoes

Serves 2

1 courgette
1 small aubergine
1 tablespoon vegetable oil
1 medium onion, chopped
1 clove garlic, finely chopped
1 small pepper, seeded and chopped
12oz/390g tin tomatoes
black pepper to taste

Slice the courgette and the aubergine. Leave to drain for 30 minutes. Rinse well and squeeze out any excess moisture. Heat the oil in a frying pan. Add the onion and garlic, and fry. Then add all the vegetables except the tomatoes and sauté for a few minutes. Add the tomatoes and season with black pepper. Cover and simmer for 30 minutes.

Winter soup

Serves 2

1 large carrot
1 large onion
2 sticks celery
½ small turnip
2 medium potatoes
½ pint/300ml vegetable stock
6 sprigs parsley
grated nutmeg to taste
ground black pepper to taste

Chop up all the vegetables and put them into a large saucepan. Add the stock and simmer for 1 hour. Just before the end of the cooking time, add the parsley. Season with grated nutmeg and black pepper.

Jamaican rice

Serves 2

1 tablespoon vegetable oil
½ large onion, sliced
½ red apple, sliced
pinch of curry powder
½ pint/300ml water
4oz/125g brown rice
1 teaspoon black treacle
1 small banana, sliced
1 tablespoon desiccated coconut

Heat the oil and sauté the onion and apple. Add the curry powder and water. Bring to the boil. Add the rice and treacle and cook until the water is absorbed and the rice is tender. Drain, and add the banana. Sprinkle the coconut on top and heat through for a moment, and then serve.

Banana special

Serves 2

2 bananas
1 small orange, juiced
1oz/30g sugar
½oz/15g polyunsaturated low-fat spread

Preheat the oven to 180°C (350°F/gas mark 4), and grease an ovenproof dish. Peel the bananas, cut them in half lengthways and place them in the dish. Pour the orange juice over the bananas and sprinkle the sugar on top. Place the low-fat spread on top of the bananas and cook for 15 minutes.

Spicy red pear

Serves 1

1 large pear
4 tablespoons red wine
ground *or* whole spices – ginger, cinnamon and cloves

Peel the pear, leaving it whole with the stalk on. Simmer in the red wine with the spices until cooked. Serve hot.

Fruit punch

Makes about 1 pint/600ml

1 pint/600ml natural (unsweetened) pineapple juice
1 banana, sliced
1 apple, chopped
1oz/30g sesame seeds
1oz/30g sunflower seeds
1oz/30g raisins
1oz/30g currants

Put all the ingredients in blender and liquidize. Keep in the refrigerator and serve chilled.

Index

abbatoirs, 9, 66–7, 86
Aboriginals Australian, 18, 86
acne, 68
addiction to food, 113–18
additives, 77–81
adrenalin, 66
advertising, 33, 42, 115, 150
aerobics, 108–9
Africa, 11, 87, 90
air travel, 13
alcohol, 71, 72, 151
alcoholism, 116, 117, 156
allergies, 3, 68
  food, 116–17
  food additives and, 81
  processed food and, 5
  to fluoride, 56–57
  to milk, 164
aluminium sulphate, 55–6
Alzheimer's disease, 55
American Journal of Diseases of Children, 124
amino acids, 16, 21, 35–8
amphetamines, 106, 115
ampicillin, 58
anaemia, 39, 47–9, 62, 69
anaesthetics, 99
aneurin, 38, 46
angina, 62
animal fats, 6
animals:
  carnivorous, 9
  cruelty to, 9–11, 86–90
  slaughtering, 9, 66–7, 86–7
anorexia nervosa, 42, 115
Anson, Admiral, 49
antibiotics, 58, 64, 166
anxiety, 69
appendicitis, 23, 62
appetite control centre, 114, 123–4, 128, 144, 147, 155, 156
apple diet, 105
arthritis, 3, 66, 74, 97, 98
artificial fabrics, 17
artificial insemination, 87
artificial sweeteners, 149
ascorbic acid, 48–9
Asia, 11
asthma, 69, 97, 99, 163
atherosclerosis, 30, 69–70
aubergines:
  Greek tomatoes, 193
Australia, 86
Aboriginals, 18

baby food, 65
bacteria:
  drug-resistant, 64
  food poisoning, 83, 84
balanced diets, 159
balloons in stomach, 108
bananas:
  banana special, 195
  Jamaican rice, 194

barbecues, 67
barley, 171
beans, 170
Belgium, 32, 65
Belinda, 136
beri-beri, 39, 46
bicycles, exercise, 108–9
biscuits, 151, 159–60
  nut biscuits, 187
blood:
  cholesterol levels, 30
  sugar levels, 122, 147–8, 149
blood pressure, 98
  see also high blood pressure
body shaping programme, 142–4
bones:
  brittle, 163
  and overweight, 111
boredom, 125–6, 127–8, 151
bowels:
  cancer, 23
  herbivores, 19
  irritable bowel syndrome, 73–4
brain:
  appetite control centre, 124–5, 129, 145, 147, 155
  blood vessels, 140–1
bran, oat, 171
Brazil, 65, 90
bread, 23, 78, 160
breakfast cereals, 160–1
breasts:
  cancer, 25, 26, 35, 62, 70
  and imagination, 141–2
breathing, 142
British Medical Journal, 40
broccoli:
  French broccoli, 184
  green chicken, 175
bronchitis, 99
buckwheat, 171
Buddhism, 11
bulimia nervosa, 115
buns, 161
burger, turkey barbecue, 177
burghul wheat:
  Russian chilli, 192
butter, 28, 163–4
Butter Information Council, 33

caffeine, 69, 72, 74
cakes, 161
calcium, 16–17, 35, 44, 50, 52–3, 164, 165
calories, 104, 148, 149, 151
cancer, 3, 70
  bowel, 23
  breast, 25, 26, 35, 62, 70
  colon, 25, 26, 62, 70
  and fat consumption, 70
  and fluoridation, 56
  and food additives, 80
  and high-protein diet, 35
  intestinal, 54

Eskimos, 68
essential fatty acids (EFAs), 30, 165
Ethiopia, 90
European Community, 163
evenings, eating in, 122–4
exercise, 34, 108–10, 153
'experts', 6
eyes, cataracts, 70

farming:
  cruelty to animals, 9–11, 85–9
  fertilizers, 54, 76–7, 90
  fish, 166–7
  meat production, 19–20, 61, 63–66
  milk production, 163–4
  nitrates pollution, 54
  pressure groups, 33
fast food chains, 13
fats, 5–6, 28–33
  and cancer, 70
  and diabetes, 71
  and gallstones, 71
  and heart disease, 69–70
  high-fat diet, 106
  low-fat diet, 106
feet, and overweight, 102
fertilizers, 54, 76–7, 90
fibre, 6, 22–25, 34, 70, 71, 72, 74, 75, 160, 161, 171
fish, 14, 15–16, 29, 165–7
  cod casserole, 178
  fish on a stick, 177
  fishcakes, 178
  fisherman's pie, 179
flavourings, 79
flies, 65
fluids, low-fluid diet, 107
fluoride, 55–7
folic acid, 47–8
food:
  addiction to, 113–18
  additives, 77–81
  allergies, 68, 71, 116–17, 163, 164
  fat content, 5–6
  'food combining', 37
  labels, 81, 150
  malnutrition, 5
  obsession with, 131–2, 148
  primitive man's diet, 18–19
food poisoning, 3, 82–4, 167, 169
free-range eggs, 78, 83, 167
French broccoli, 184
fridges, 82–4
frozen food, 82–3
fructose, 27
fruit, 8, 167
  contamination, 76–7
  organic, 75
  skins, 148
  sugar content, 27
fruit punch, 196
fruitarianism, 14, 88
fruity yoghurt, 188
frying, 150
fungicides, 76
fungus infections, 97
fur coats, 17

gall bladder disease, 71, 99
gallstones, 23, 63, 71
gastric ulcers, 75

gastrointestinal disorders, 82
germanium, 42–3
glucose, 25, 149
glucose sweets, 147–8
goat's milk, 164
golden vegetable parcels, 183
gout, 29, 63, 66, 71, 97
grains, 170–1
grapefruit diet, 105
Greek tomatoes, 193
green chicken, 175
growth hormones, 64–5
guilt, 125–6
gum disease, 75

haddock:
  fisherman's pie, 179
haemorrhoids, 63
hay fever, 68
headaches, 72, 117, 140
heart:
  body shaping programme, 143
  and overweight, 98, 99
heart disease, 3
  fats and, 29, 30–1, 69–70
  high-protein diet, 35
  meat and, 62–3
  overweight and, 97
  processed food and, 5
  sugar and, 26
herbicides, 76
herbivores, 18–9
hernias, 97, 99
high blood pressure, 3, 5, 29, 63, 69, 72–3, 97
high-carbohydrate diet, 107
high-fat diet, 106
high-protein diet, 35, 107
Hinduism, 11
holidays, 12–13
honey, 25
hormones:
  fish farming, 166–7
  meat production, 63–5
  milk production, 164
  residues in drinking water, 58, 60
hot devilled eggs, 185
hotels, 13
hotpots:
  Portuguese, 191
  vegetable, 188
Humphrey, Senator Hubert, 89
hunger pangs, 147–8
hygiene:
  abbatoirs, 66–7
  in kitchens, 83
Hygienists, 14
hyperactivity, 80

illnesses, 67–74
imagination, 137–42
  body shaping programme, 142–4
India, 89
indigestion, 3, 63, 73
infections, 73
insecticides, 76
insomnia, 73
insulin, 25, 99, 149
intestines:
  cancer, 54
  surgical treatment of overweight, 108
'intrinsic factor', 48